Paediatric Advanced Life Support
A Practical Guide

Philip Jevon BSc(Hons) RN PGCE
Resuscitation Training Officer, Manor Hospital, Walsall, UK

Consultant editors

Kirsti Soanes BSc(Hons) RGN RSCN
Lead Nurse, Children's Accident and Emergency Department, University
Hospitals of Leicester NHS Trust, Leicester, UK

Kathleen Berry FRCP(c), FRCPCH, FFAEM
Consultant in Paediatric Accident and Emergency Medicine, Birmingham
Children's Hospital, Birmingham, UK

Gale A. Pearson MB BS MRCP FRCPCH
Head of Specialty, Paediatric Intensive Care Unit, Birmingham Children's
Hospital, Birmingham, UK

Foreword by

Tom Beattie MB MSc FRCS(Ed) FFAEM DCH
Consultant in Accident and Emergency Care, Royal Hospital for
Sick Children, Edinburgh, UK

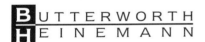

BUTTERWORTH
HEINEMANN

EDINBURGH LONDON NEW YORK OXFORD PHILADELPHIA ST LOUIS SYDNEY TORONTO 2004

BUTTERWORTH-HEINEMANN
An imprint of Elsevier Limited

First published 2004
  Reprinted 2004

ISBN 0 7506 5599 2

British Library Cataloguing in Publication Data
A catalogue record for this book is available from the British Library

Library of Congress Cataloging in Publication Data
A catalog record for this book is available from the Library of Congress

Notice
Medical knowledge is constantly changing. Stantard safety
precautions must be followed, but as new research and clinical
experience broaden our knowledge, changes in treatment and drug
therapy may become necessary or appropriate. Readers are advised to
check the most current product information provided by the
manufacturer of each drug to be administered to verify the
recommended dose, the method and duration of administration, and
contraindications. It is the responsibility of the practitioner, relying on
experience and knowledge of the patient, to determine dosages and
the best treatment for each individual patient. Neither the Publisher
nor the author assumes any liability for any injury and/or damage to
persons or property arising from this publication.

The Publisher

 your source for books,
journals and multimedia
in the health sciences
www.elsevierhealth.com

The
publisher's
policy is to use
**paper manufactured
from sustainable forests**

Printed in China

Paediatric Advanced Life Support

Cover image courtesy of Cook Incorporated,
Bloomington, Indiana, USA.

For Butterworth Heinemann:

Senior Commissioning Editor: Ninette Premdas
Project Development Manager: Mairi McCubbin
Project Manager: Ailsa Laing
Designer: George Ajayi
Illustrations Manager: Bruce Hogarth
Indexer: Dr Laurence Errington

Contents

Foreword

There can be few more stressful situations than to be presented with a desperately ill or dying infant or child. Thankfully such circumstances are relatively rare in the developed world, although they still remain much more frequent elsewhere. Though a rare occurrence, clinicians and healthcare workers will inevitably be presented with children in extremis. The relative frequency will depend on the field of practice. A family practitioner in an urban setting might expect to see one critically ill child every ten to fifteen years, while encountering tens of mild to moderately ill children weekly. The emergency paediatrician will see several hundred critically ill children annually. The expectations of and from each practitioner will vary greatly, and each perspective will be different. Despite being at the frontline for more years than I care to dwell on, I still get a frisson of unease when the crash box announces yet another critically ill child is nigh!

The role of first responders in these critical situations is to firstly recognize the urgency of the situation, and then to summon experienced help. While senior help is awaited, simple measures can and should be instituted. Especially important in the paediatric setting is the maintenance of a clear airway and oxygenation. Once senior help arrives, bringing with it such skills as expertise in airway care, skill at intravenous access and leadership, definitive resuscitation can begin. Even so, the outcome of out-of-hospital cardiac arrest is dismal. Most will die, and those few survivors are likely to have neurological impairment.

Thus, a structured, step-wise approach is paramount. It only comes from practicing in a well-ordered system. The system is as important as the practice!

The improvement in mortality from paediatric critical care situations has been well documented in the UK since the introduction of structured life-support courses in the early 1990s. These courses highlight the need for recognition of the sick child and provide a framework within which appropriate care can be delivered. The principles of 'back to safety' are paramount. Prior to this several authors reported on the unpreparedness of all grades of staff to deal with acute paediatric emergencies.

It is also well documented that failure to revise or practice skills learnt from these courses leads to a loss of skill. Therefore, once trained, practitioners must endeavour to maintain practice at as high a level as is compatible with the likely need to practice. Retention of motor skills is important – practice makes perfect – however theory and baseline knowledge are equally important.

To this end, this book by Phil Jevon and his colleagues provides one mechanism for maintaining these skills. As a text it incorporates up-to-date concepts of the structure and organization for Paediatric Emergency and Early Critical Care Management. The most recent guidelines available have been promulgated as a means to providing optimal care in the emergency and cardiac arrest situation. These guidelines are, however, just that – a guide to best practice. Much of what is taught is derived from good science. However, the remainder is based on past practice, opinion and history. That is not to say it is wrong; it merely supports current practice as the best we can do at the present time. Readers should attempt to identify scientifically-based practice from the opinion and use this as a stimulus to question how we might do better. It would be pleasing to find that this text appears as future editions, containing better and more effective strategies for dealing with critical paediatric illness.

What is particularly pleasing is the emphasis on the preparation for cardiac arrest, a topic that is often neglected. Similarly, the structure for paediatric resuscitation training and the equipment available for training is also very useful. This latter is an oft-neglected area. Resuscitation is an extremely practical process, albeit one requiring a modicum of supporting theory. Medical texts tend to concentrate on the clinical content in isolation. Without discussion of the means for knowledge transfer and the arrangements for dissemination, resuscitation texts can be sterile.

This text is extremely readable and accessible. It follows the continuum of resuscitation circumstances and procedures in a logical sequence, akin to that which might well apply in real life. The inclusion of audit and documentation demonstrates the affinity the authors have with real-world situations. Ethical concerns regarding resuscitation are well covered, as is bereavement. These are areas that I personally find difficult, and it is good to find these areas addressed. Above all the plethora of useful contacts and references throughout provide a resource for further study.

The junior nurse picking it up for the first time will not be overawed by the content. The senior clinician will find a basis for further research, aided by the comprehensive references attached to each chapter. Whether as a single text for learning or a resource to be tapped for revision, there is something for everyone.

Dr Tom Beattie
Edinburgh 2003

Acknowledgements

I would like to thank Kathleen Berry, Gale Pearson and Kirsti Soanes for their help and advice. Kirsti Soanes also wrote the majority of the chapter on bereavement (Chapter 12).

Sharon Worth RN, formally trainee solicitor at Mills-Reeve Solicitors, assisted with the ethical and legal issues chapter in my book *Resuscitation in Pregnancy: a practical approach* (2001), from which some text has been reproduced in Chapter 14 of this book

Many thanks to: Gale Pearson for providing me with Fig. 11.6, BMJ Publishing for granting me permission to reproduce Box 10.1 and the Oakley Chart, Laerdal Medical for granting me permission to reproduce their ECG traces, Aurum Pharmaceuticals for granting me permission to reproduce their artwork of the BLS, ALS and anaphylaxis algorithms, Cook Incorporated, Bloomington, IN, USA for Fig. 8.5 and the cover image, and the Advanced life Support Group in Manchester for photographs and boxes from their APLS Manual.

John Hamilton, Medical Photography at the Manor Hospital in Walsall, helped with the photographs and Elaine Walton, Resuscitation Officer Manor Hospital, Walsall kindly agreed to be the 'rescuer' in the CPR photographs.

My thanks to Birmingham Children's Hospital for granting me permission to reproduce their modified Paediatric Coma Score chart and the front cover of their bereavement booklet.

Chapter 1

Overview of paediatric advanced life support

Introduction

Paediatric advanced life support (PALS) includes the knowledge and skills necessary to identify and effectively treat infants and children who have potential respiratory or circulatory failure, and to provide the appropriate treatment in the event of a paediatric cardiac arrest.

The aim of this chapter is to provide an overview of PALS.

Objectives

At the end of the chapter the reader will be able to:

- discuss the causes of cardiac arrest in childhood
- outline the pathophysiology of paediatric cardiac arrest
- discuss the survival rates following paediatric resuscitation
- outline the provision of a resuscitation service in hospital
- discuss the recommended standards for the reception of critically ill children in hospital
- discuss the recommended general standards for all critically ill children.

Causes of cardiac arrest in childhood

The exact causes of cardiac arrest in childhood vary from study to study depending on whether the arrest occurred in the in-hospital setting (Lewis *et al.*, 1983; Gillis *et al.*, 1986; Innes *et al.*, 1993) or the out-of-hospital setting (Eisenberg *et al.*, 1983; O'Rourke *et al.*, 1986). The commonest causes will result in respiratory or circulatory insufficiency leading to cardiorespiratory failure (Bingham, 1996).

According to the Office of National Statistics (1998), the highest death rates in childhood occur during the first year of life, particularly the first month (Table 1.1).

Causes of death in childhood vary according to age. The most common causes are:

- *newborn period:* congenital abnormalities and factors associated with prematurity
- *1 month to 1 year:* cot death, infection and congenital abnormality
- *from 1 year:* trauma.

Table 1.1   Death rates in childhood

Age group	Number of deaths (rate)		
	1991 (E&W)	1998 (E&W)	1998 (Australia)
0–28 days	3052 (4.4)	24189 (3.8)	842 (5.02)
4–52 weeks	2106 (3.0)	1207 (1.9)	410
1–4 years	993 (36)	722 (28)	347
5–14 years	1165 (19)	897 (13)	376
1–14 years	2158 (24)	1619 (17)	723 (19.7)

The rate for under ones is per 1000 population and for over ones per 100 000 population
England and Wales, 1991 and 1998 Office of National Statistics (ONS) Australia 1998 (from
ALSG, 2001, with kind permission)

Pathophysiology of cardiac arrest

There are three basic mechanisms of paediatric cardiac arrest: asystole; pulseless electrical activity (PEA – formally known as electromechanical dissociation or EMD); and ventricular fibrillation (VF). Pulseless ventricular tachycardia (VT) is another mechanism, but is usually classified with VF because the causes and treatment are similar.

Asystole

Asystole (Fig. 1.1) is the most common presenting rhythm in paediatric cardiac arrests (Sirbaugh et al., 1999; Young and Seidel, 1999). It is the final common pathway of respiratory or circulatory failure (Zideman and Spearpoint, 1999). Prolonged severe hypoxia and acidosis lead to progressive bradycardia and asystole (ALSG, 2001). The most common cause is hypoxia and the most effective treatment is to establish a clear airway and effective ventilation (Zideman, 1997).

Management of asystole is less commonly successful than when the rhythm is VF (Dieckmann and Vardis, 1995), but survival to discharge has been reported (Spearpoint, 2002).

PEA

PEA (formally called electromechanical dissociation or EMD) is a term used to signify the features of cardiac arrest associated with a normal (or near normal) ECG. The diagnosis is made on clinical grounds by the combination of the absence of a cardiac output with an ECG rhythm on the monitor that would normally be associated with a good cardiac output.

The causes of PEA can be classified into one of two broad categories:

Primary PEA   There is failure of excitation contraction coupling in the cardiac myocytes resulting in profound loss of cardiac output. Causes include hypoxia, poisoning, e.g. due to beta-blockers, calcium channel blockers or toxins, and electrolyte disturbance (hyperkalaemia or hypocalcaemia).

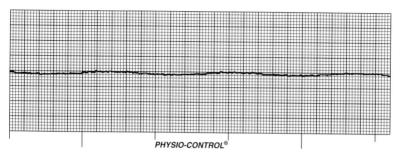

PHYSIO-CONTROL®

Fig. 1.1   Asystole.

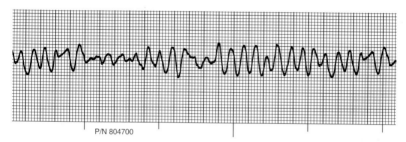

P/N 804700

Fig. 1.2   Ventricular fibrillation.

Secondary PEA   There is a mechanical barrier to ventricular filling or ejection. Causes include hypovolaemia, cardiac tamponade and tension pneumothorax.

In all cases treatment is directed towards the cause.

VF/VT

VF/VT is uncommon in children (Zideman and Spearpoint, 1999; Spearpoint, 2002). However, clinical situations when it may occur include after cardiac surgery, cardiomyopathy, congenital heart disease, hypothermia and drug intoxication.

In VF (Fig. 1.2) the ECG displays a bizarre irregular waveform, apparently random in both frequency and amplitude, reflecting disorganized electrical activity in the myocardium. It is an eminently treatable arrhythmia, but the only effective treatment is early defibrillation and the likelihood of success is crucially dependent upon timing (Jevon, 2002).

Conditions for defibrillation are optimal for as little as 90 seconds after the onset of the rhythm, and the chances of success fall by about 10% with every minute that treatment is delayed (Colquhoun and Jevon, 2000). Untreated VF will inevitably deteriorate into asystole as myocardial energy reserves and oxygen are exhausted; successful CPR at this late stage is almost impossible (Colquhoun and Jevon, 2000).

Survival rates following paediatric resuscitation

Paediatric cardiac arrest is rarely caused by a primary cardiac problem. In addition it is rarely a sudden event (Klitzener, 1995). It is often the end result of progressive deterioration in respiratory and circulatory function (American Academy of Pediatrics, 2000). If cardiac arrest ensues, the prognosis is dismal (O'Rourke, 1986). Survival rates of patients in asystole are reported to be as low as 3% (Zaritsky *et al.*, 1987).

The early recognition and aggressive management of respiratory or cardiac insufficiency (Ch. 3) aimed at preventing deterioration to cardiac arrest are the key to improving survival without neurological deficit in seriously ill children (Zideman and Spearpoint, 1999).

Prompt resuscitation in the event of a respiratory arrest is associated with a favourable outcome, particularly if it is detected and treated before cardiac arrest (Lewis *et al.*, 1983; Innes *et al.*, 1993). Survival rates of > 50% have been reported for respiratory arrests (Zaritsky *et al.*, 1987; Spearpoint, 2002).

Provision of a resuscitation service in hospital

Hospitals have a duty of care to ensure that an effective resuscitation service is provided and all appropriate staff are adequately trained and regularly updated to a level compatible with their expected degree of competence.

The Resuscitation Council (UK) in their report 'Cardiopulmonary resuscitation guidance for clinical practice and training in hospitals' (Resuscitation Council (UK), 2001) has made a number of recommendations in respect of the provision of a resuscitation service in hospital. Each will now be discussed.

Resuscitation committee

Every hospital should have a resuscitation committee, which meets on a regular basis. It should comprise at least five members, who have an active interest in CPR, for example:

- physician
- resuscitation officer
- anaesthetist (or practitioner with anaesthetic experience)
- representatives from appropriate departments, e.g. A&E, paediatrics
- nurse
- junior doctor.

The committee should advise on the paediatric cardiac arrest team, resuscitation equipment and resuscitation training equipment. It should ensure that European Resuscitation Council guidelines for paediatric advanced life support (2001) (Fig. 1.3) are implemented effectively and that there are adequate financial resources available for CPR and resuscitation training.

Resuscitation training officer

Every hospital should have at least one person responsible for resuscitation training, ideally a designated full-time resuscitation training officer (RTO).

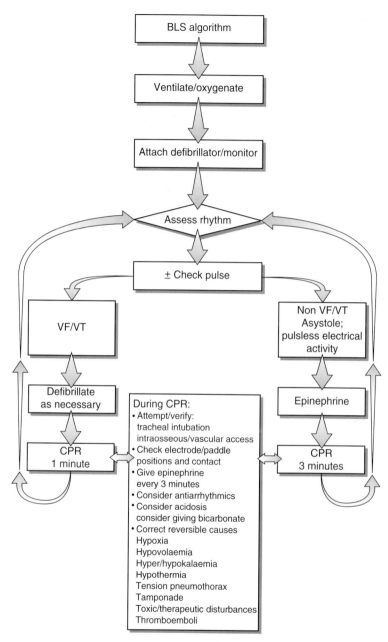

Fig. 1.3 European Resuscitation Council paediatric advanced life support algorithm 2001 (reproduced with permission of Aurum Pharmaceuticals).

The RTO should be a member of the resuscitation committee and should be accountable to a nominated doctor on the committee. The RTO may also be accountable to a senior nurse or the Training Department manager.

The RTO should ideally be a Resuscitation Council (UK) ALS instructor. He or she should have adequate training facilities and CPR training equipment. Secretarial support should be provided.

Responsibilities of the RTO include:

- providing adequate resuscitation training for relevant hospital personnel
- ensuring that all resuscitation equipment for clinical use is regularly checked and maintained to an appropriate standard – although this is often delegated to other staff, the RTO should nevertheless undertake regular audits to ensure it is being done
- auditing CPR attempts using a common template, e.g. Utstein
- attending CPR attempts and providing feedback to team members
- coordinating participation in CPR-related trials
- keeping abreast of current CPR guidelines.

Resuscitation training

Hospital staff should receive regular resuscitation training appropriate to their level and expected clinical responsibilities. This is discussed further in Chapter 15.

Paediatric resuscitation team

The composition of the paediatric resuscitation team should be determined by the resuscitation committee. The team leader should be someone with expertise and training in paediatric resuscitation. Although at least one member of the team should be trained in paediatric advanced life support, all staff who are regularly responsible for paediatric resuscitation should be encouraged to undertake a nationally recognized course in paediatric resuscitation (see pp. 160–161). The paediatric team should be alerted following local protocols; this usually involves dialling 222 and informing the hospital switchboard of the paediatric arrest and its location.

Resuscitation equipment

The resuscitation committee is responsible for advising on resuscitation equipment, which will largely be dependent upon local requirements and facilities. Ideally it should be standardized throughout the hospital. Resuscitation equipment is discussed in detail in the next chapter.

'Do not attempt resuscitation' orders

Every hospital should have a 'do not attempt resuscitation' policy, which should be based on national guidelines (BMA *et al.*, 2001) (Ch. 14).

Transfer of the child and post-resuscitation care

Complete recovery from a cardiac arrest is rarely immediate and the return of spontaneous circulation is just the start, not the end, of the resuscitation attempt. The immediate post-resuscitation period is characterized by high dependency and clinical instability with some children requiring transfer to a paediatric intensive therapy unit (ITU). The principles of transfer of the child and post-resuscitation care are discussed in Chapter 11.

Auditing and reporting standards

The resuscitation committee should ensure that all resuscitation attempts are audited, ideally using a nationally recognized template (Utstein). The audit should include the availability and performance of the paediatric resuscitation team members, the standard and reliability of resuscitation equipment and the on-going management of the child in the post-resuscitation phase. Audit is discussed in more detail in Chapter 13.

Standards for the reception of critically ill children in hospital

The Paediatric Intensive Care Society (PICS) recommends in its 'Standards Document 2001' the following standards for the reception of critically ill children:

Applicability

- All hospitals potentially admitting children who are, or who may become, critically ill must be able to resuscitate and stabilize them.
- Only A&E departments that are on the same hospital site as inpatient paediatric facilities should accept children but all hospitals should have in place a protocol for use in the event of a critically ill (or potentially critically ill) child presenting to them.
- All hospitals which have on-site inpatient paediatric facilities must be able to receive, assess, resuscitate and stabilize the child and immediately refer to the HDU or paediatric intensive care team on site or have the ability to initiate and maintain paediatric intensive care until the retrieval team arrives.

Environment and support for parents and children

- There must be compliance with the published guidance for A&E departments in relation to children.
- There must be a child and family focused environment with audiovisual separation from adult patients.
- There must be parental access to the child at all times except when this is not in the interests of the child. Written guidelines must be in place.
- There must be information available to the parents on the child's condition, care plan and retrieval (if necessary).
- There must be access to support services, e.g. chaplain and social workers (see General standards for all critically ill children, below).

Medical staffing

- Trusts must recruit a consultant with recognized training in paediatric A&E, to be responsible for the protocols, assessment and management of the critically ill child within each A&E department that accepts children.

- All A&E departments must have a named consultant with responsibility for protocols relating to the management of critically ill children.
- It is essential that there is 24-hour on-site cover by medical staff and always a doctor on duty with APLS/PALS or equivalent training in the reception areas/amongst the receiving staff.

Access/provision of advice between lead centre and referring hospital

- Advice must always be available from the local paediatric medical in-patient unit and the lead centre for paediatric intensive care.
- An agreed protocol should be in place for accessing advice 24 hours a day. The protocol must be discussed, agreed and regularly reviewed by all the hospitals in the catchment area including the lead centre and should conform to the standards for referral to paediatric intensive care.

Nurse staffing

- There should be a senior nurse (RSCN on Part 8 of the NMC register or Diploma/Degree Nurse (Child) on Part 15 of the NMC register) responsible for ensuring that the care of children is appropriate and undertaken in the correct environment. This nurse must ensure that there is ongoing training for the nurses in APLS/PALS skills and good liaison arrangements in place with hospital and community paediatric services.
- There should be at least one qualified nurse on duty at all times with APLS/PALS or equivalent skills.
- Nurse-led minor injury units should not look after acutely ill children. However all shifts at such a unit must include a staff member with basic paediatric airway skills, training in paediatric resuscitation, access to locally agreed protocols for the management of an acutely ill child and good liaison with the lead centre.

Equipment and facilities

- There should be a separate (with audiovisual separation from facilities used for adults), designated and equipped area for the resuscitation and stabilization of critically ill children of all ages.
- Critically ill children awaiting retrieval should be looked after in a high-dependency area, the location and facilities of which should be known by, and agreed with, the retrieval team.
- There should be access to appropriate support services (e.g. chaplain, and social services) and facilities for parents, including a quiet room.

Quality and management of services

- There must be a system within the hospital alerting appropriate staff to the arrival of a critically ill child.

- There must be protocols in place covering the resuscitation, stabiliza-tion, transfer, admission, discharge and treatment of all major condi-tions for use in the A&E department. These need to be developed in conjunction with the paediatricians, the lead centre and other appropri-ate specialties.
- A critical incident reporting system must be in place as part of the clin-ical governance audit system.
- Cases referred on for intensive care must be subject to quality assurance and audit.

General standards for all critically ill children

The Paediatric Intensive Care Society (PICS) recommends in its 'Standards Document 2001' the following general standards for all critically ill children:

The interests of the child

- In all actions concerning children, the interests of the child shall be the paramount consideration.
- The interests of children of all abilities, from all groups and socio-economic backgrounds should be valued equally.

Children are different

- Staffing facilities, equipment and accommodation should be appro-priate to the needs of children and separate from those provided for adults.
- Children under 16 years of age should not be treated on adult wards except under extenuating circumstances (e.g. obstetric conditions).
- All staff should be trained to work with children and should be familiar with their needs.
- Each child should be admitted under the care of a consultant paediatric specialist.
- Each hospital should have a named consultant paediatric specialist with an administrative responsibility for critically ill children.

The child's right to be heard

- The consent of the parent/carer should wherever possible be obtained to treat children under 16 years of age. Where a child has sufficient under-standing and intelligence to give or withhold consent, a note should be made in the medical records of the factors taken into account.
- Children should receive such information about all aspects of their diag-nosis and treatment as is appropriate to their age, understanding, com-munication ability, and language. 'Play techniques' should be used where appropriate.

The importance of the family

- Adequate facilities should be available to enable parents/carers to stay with their child and help with care for them in the location where the child is treated.
- Visiting arrangements should allow contact with other family members such as siblings.
- Parents/carers should be able to have access to their child, except where this is not in the interests of the child. Guidelines for these circumstances must be in place and implemented.
- All professionals must be trained in the skills necessary to work effectively with parents/carers.
- All those with parental responsibility should be fully informed to enable them to be involved in making decisions about the care of their children.
- The views of parents, carers and children should influence the planning of services.
- Interpretation services for children and families of different cultural and ethnic backgrounds should be routinely available 24 hours a day.

Protecting children from harm

- All staff have a duty to protect children.
- Policies and procedures should be in place to reduce the risk of harm. These should include safe procedures for the selection and training of staff working with children, procedures for the prevention of abuse and hospital security.
- Where abuse is suspected, agencies should follow the procedures for working together produced by their area child protection committee.
- Procedures should be in place for investigating and reporting untoward incidents.
- Health commissioners and providers should be aware of what is considered best practice, and have access to sources of information and advice on effective healthcare.
- A system of critical incident reporting should be in place.

Provision of the service

- Because of the nature of the specialty and the nature of medical and nursing training, many aspects of the care of critically ill children must be delivered by senior nursing and medical (consultant) staff. Many aspects of these standards are written with that in mind.
- The admission of children to high-dependency and intensive-care areas must be under the supervision of duty consultants who if they are not personally present should be expected to review the patient soon after admission.

Summary

PALS includes the knowledge and skills necessary to identify and effectively treat infants and children who have potential respiratory or circulatory failure, and to provide the appropriate treatment in the event of a paediatric cardiac arrest.

The importance of the early diagnosis and aggressive treatment of respiratory or circulatory insufficiency has been discussed. In addition the recommended standards for the reception of critically ill children in hospital and the general standards for all critically ill children have been highlighted.

Chapter 2

Resuscitation equipment

Introduction

A speedy response is essential in the event of a paediatric cardiac arrest. Procedures should be in place to ensure that all the essential equipment is immediately available, accessible and in good working order. A carefully set out and fully stocked cardiac arrest trolley is paramount.

The aim of this chapter is to discuss the provision of resuscitation equipment for paediatric resuscitation.

Objectives

At the end of this chapter the reader will be able to:

- list the resuscitation equipment required for paediatric resuscitation
- list the aids available to estimate paediatric drug doses and equipment sizes
- discuss the routine checking of resuscitation equipment
- discuss the checking of resuscitation equipment following use.

Resuscitation equipment required for paediatric resuscitation

The following is a suggested list of resuscitation equipment required for paediatric resuscitation:

Airway and breathing

- Pocket mask with oxygen port
- Self-inflating resuscitation bags (500 ml and 1500 ml) with oxygen reservoir and oxygen tubing
- Selection of clear facemasks
- Oropharyngeal airways – various sizes
- Rigid wide-bore (Yankauer) suckers
- Tracheal suction catheters – various sizes
- Tracheal tubes – full range of sizes
- Gum elastic bougie
- Lubricating jelly
- Laryngoscopes × 2 – Miller 1 (straight), Macintosh 1, 2 and 3 blades
- Spare laryngoscope bulbs and batteries
- 1 inch ribbon gauze/tape
- Scissors
- Syringe – 20 ml

- Non-rebreathe oxygen mask with reservoir bag
- Oxygen cylinder(s) and cylinder key.

Circulation

- Intravenous cannulae – selection
- Intraosseous infusion needles
- Hypodermic needles – various sizes
- Syringes – various sizes
- Cannula fixing dressings and tapes
- Seldinger wire central line kit
- Non-Seldinger central venous cannulae
- Intravenous giving sets
- 0.9% sodium chloride 500-ml bags.

Drugs (Fig. 2.1)

- Epinephrine (adrenaline) 1 mg (1 : 10 000) × 4
- Atropine 3 mg × 1
- Amiodarone 300 mg × 1
- Sodium bicarbonate 8.4% – 50 ml × 1

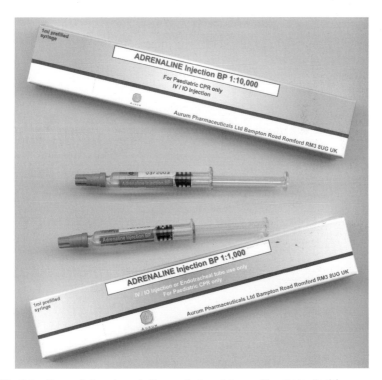

Fig. 2.1   Resuscitation drugs (with permission of Aurum Pharmaceuticals).

- Calcium chloride 13.24% – 10 ml × 2
- Normal saline 10-ml ampoules × 10
- Naloxone 400 µg × 2
- Epinephrine (adrenaline) 1 : 1000 × 2
- Magnesium sulphate 50% solution 2 g (4 ml) × 1
- Glucose 10% 500 ml × 1.

Additional items

- Paediatric resuscitation chart or tape (or similar)
- ECG electrodes
- Defibrillation gel pads
- Clock

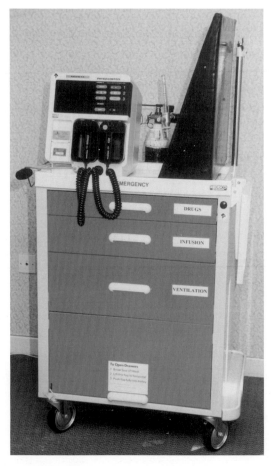

Fig. 2.2 Cardiac arrest trolley.

- Gloves/goggles/aprons
- A sliding sheet or similar device should be available for safer handling
- Pulse oximeter.

The resuscitation equipment should be stored on a standard cardiac arrest trolley (Fig. 2.2). It should be spacious, sturdy, easily accessible and mobile. Every trolley should be identically stocked to avoid confusion. A defibrillator (with paediatric paddles) should also be immediately available.

Although piped or wall oxygen and suction should always be used when available, portable suction devices and oxygen should still be at hand, either on or adjacent to the cardiac arrest trolley. Other items that the cardiac arrest team should have immediate access to include a stethoscope, ECG machine, blood pressure measuring device, pulse oximeter, blood gas syringes and a device for verifying correct tracheal tube placement, e.g. oesophageal detector device.

Aids to estimating paediatric drug doses and equipment sizes

Estimating drug doses and equipment sizes is important when managing a paediatric cardiac arrest (Zideman and Spearpoint, 1999). Several aids are currently available which help with these calculations including the Walsall Paediatric Resuscitation Chart, the Oakley Chart, the Broselow/Hinkle Paediatric Emergency System and the Paediatric Resuscitation and Emergency Management (PREM) System. It is important to become familiar with one specific system.

Walsall Paediatric Resuscitation Chart

The Walsall Paediatric Resuscitation Chart (Fig. 2.3) has been designed based on recommendations by Burke and Bowden (1993). A recent study favours the simple and clear approach this chart has adopted, with all the drug doses recommended in millilitres using standard concentrations.

The Oakley Chart

The Oakley chart (Fig. 2.4) was first proposed in 1988 (Oakley, 1988). It was recognized at that time that a simple, versatile and readily available reference chart was required for paediatric resuscitation because of the variation in size of infants and children and the comparative infrequency of paediatric cardiopulmonary arrests. The chart was revised in 1993, reflecting the new Resuscitation Council (UK) guidelines for paediatric advanced life support (Oakley *et al.*, 1993).

The Broselow/Hinkle Paediatric Emergency System

The Broselow/Hinkle Paediatric Emergency System (Fig. 2.5) provides a fast, accurate method for the selection of emergency equipment and drug

NB. ALL DRUG DOSES ARE IN MILLILITRES (MLS), I/V OR INTRAOSSEOUS UNLESS OTHERWISE STATED.

AGE		MONTHS		YEARS					
		3	6	1	3.5	6	10	13	14
WEIGHT (KG)		5	7	10	15	20	30	40	50
ADRENALINE/ 1:10,000 EPINEPHERINE	Initial	0.5	0.7	1	1.5	2	3	4	5
ADRENALINE/ 1:1,000 EPINEPHERINE	Subsequent or initial endotracheal	0.5	0.7	1	1.5	2	3	4	5
SODIUM BICARBONATE 4.2%		10	14	20	30	40	60	80	100
CALCIUM CHLORIDE 10%		0.5	0.7	1	1.5	2	3	4	5
DEXTROSE 10%		25	35	50	75	100	150	200	250
LIGNOCAINE/LIDOCAINE 1%		0.5	0.7	1	1.5	2	3	4	5
INITIAL FLUID BOLUS IN SHOCK		100	140	200	300	400	600	800	1000
ET TUBE SIZE (MM) (Internal diameter)		3.5	4	4	5	6	6.5	7.5	7.5
ET TUBE SIZE (CM) (Length)		10	11	12	14	16	17	18	19
INITIAL DC DEFIBRILLATION (J)		10	15	20	30	40	60	80	100

Fig. 2.3   Walsall Paediatric Resuscitation Chart.

doses. First the child's length is measured and assigned one of the seven colour ranges. A coordinated colour pack is taken from the Broselow/ Hinkle system. The full system comprises a manual resuscitation system, intubation modules, oxygen delivery modules, i.v. delivery modules, intraosseous access modules and blood pressure cuffs.

PREM

The Paediatric Resuscitation and Emergency Management (PREM) System provides guidelines for the management of paediatric emergencies.

Endotracheal tube

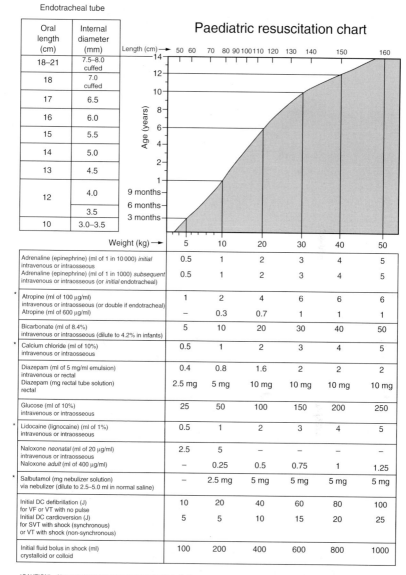

Weight (kg) →	5	10	20	30	40	50
Adrenaline (epinephrine) (ml of 1 in 10 000) *initial* intravenous or intraosseous	0.5	1	2	3	4	5
Adrenaline (epinephrine) (ml of 1 in 1000) *subsequent* intravenous or intraosseous (or *initial* endotracheal)	0.5	1	2	3	4	5
* Atropine (ml of 100 µg/ml) intravenous or intraosseous (or double if endotracheal)	1	2	4	6	6	6
Atropine (ml of 600 µg/ml)	–	0.3	0.7	1	1	1
Bicarbonate (ml of 8.4%) intravenous or intraosseous (dilute to 4.2% in infants)	5	10	20	30	40	50
* Calcium chloride (ml of 10%) intravenous or intraosseous	0.5	1	2	3	4	5
Diazepam (ml of 5 mg/ml emulsion) intravenous or rectal	0.4	0.8	1.6	2	2	2
Diazepam (mg rectal tube solution) rectal	2.5 mg	5 mg	10 mg	10 mg	10 mg	10 mg
Glucose (ml of 10%) intravenous or intraosseous	25	50	100	150	200	250
* Lidocaine (lignocaine) (ml of 1%) intravenous or intraosseous	0.5	1	2	3	4	5
Naloxone *neonatal* (ml of 20 µg/ml) intravenous or intraosseous	2.5	5	–	–	–	–
Naloxone *adult* (ml of 400 µg/ml)	–	0.25	0.5	0.75	1	1.25
* Salbutamol (mg nebulizer solution) via nebulizer (dilute to 2.5–5.0 ml in normal saline)	–	2.5 mg	5 mg	5 mg	5 mg	5 mg
Initial DC defibrillation (J) for VF or VT with no pulse	10	20	40	60	80	100
Initial DC cardioversion (J) for SVT with shock (synchronous) or VT with shock (non-synchronous)	5	5	10	15	20	25
Initial fluid bolus in shock (ml) crystalloid or colloid	100	200	400	600	800	1000

*CAUTION!   Non-standard drug concentrations may be available:
Use Atropine 100 µg/ml or prepare by diluting 1 mg to 10 ml or 600 µg to 6 ml in normal saline.
Note that 1 ml of calcium chloride 10% is equivalent to 3 ml of calcium gluconate 10%.
Use lidocaine (lignocaine) (without adrenaline (epinephrine)) 1% or give twice the volume of 0.5%. Give half the volume of 2% or
dilute appropriately.
Salbutamol may also be given by slow intravenous injection (4–6 µg/kg), but beware of the different concentraions available
(e.g. 50 and 500 µg/ml).

Fig. 2.4   The Oakley Chart reproduced from ALSG, 1999 (with kind permission of BMJ Books).

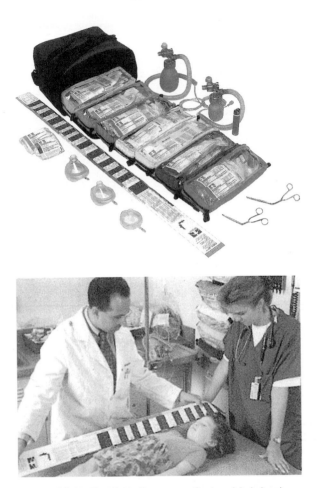

Fig. 2.5 Broselow/Hinkle Paediatric Emergency System (vital signs).

It comprises four components, designed to be used together in a complete system:

- an A4 manual for the resuscitation room
- A5 pocket-sized manuals for those responsible for paediatric resuscitation and emergency management
- drug dosage flipchart
- weight range tape.

Routine checking of resuscitation equipment

Resuscitation equipment should be checked daily by each ward or department with responsibility for the resuscitation trolley (Resuscitation Council (UK), 2001b).

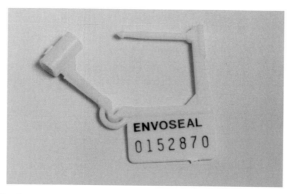

Fig. 2.6   Cardiac arrest trolley seal.

A system for daily documented checks of the equipment inventory should be in place. Some cardiac arrest trolleys can be 'sealed' with a numbered seal (Fig. 2.6) after being checked. Once the contents have been checked, the trolley can then be sealed and the seal number documented by the person who has checked the trolley. The advantage of this system is that an unbroken seal, together with the same seal number last recorded, signifies the trolley has not been opened since it was last checked and sealed. The equipment inventory should therefore be complete. A broken seal or an unrecorded seal number suggests the inventory may not be complete, hence a complete check is then required. The seal can easily be broken if the trolley needs to be opened.

Expiry dates should be checked, e.g. drugs, fluids, ECG electrodes, defibrillation pads. Laryngoscopes, including batteries and bulbs, should also be checked to ensure good working order. Each self-inflating bag should be checked to ensure that there are no leaks and that the rim of the facemask is adequately inflated.

The defibrillator should be checked on a daily basis following the manufacturer's recommendations. This usually will involve charging up and discharging the shock into the defibrillator. It is recommended that advice is sought from a member of the Electrobiomedical Engineers' (EBME) Department or from the manufacturer's representative regarding how to undertake this. In addition, most defibrillators need to be plugged into the mains to ensure that the battery is fully charged in the event of use.

Manufacturers usually recommend that ECG electrodes should be stored in their original packaging until immediately prior to use. However, the policy at some hospitals is to leave them attached to the defibrillator leads. They should therefore be checked to ensure that the gel is moist, not dry. If they are dry, they should be replaced.

All mechanical equipment, e.g. defibrillator, suction machine, should be inspected and serviced on a regular basis by the EBME Department following the manufacturer's recommendations.

Checking resuscitation equipment following use

Checking of resuscitation equipment following use should be a specifically delegated responsibility. As well as the routine checks identified above, any disposable equipment used should be replaced and reusable equipment, e.g. self-inflating bag, cleaned following local infection control procedures and manufacturer's recommendations. Any difficulties with equipment encountered during resuscitation should be documented and reported to relevant personnel.

Summary

This chapter has made suggestions for what resuscitation equipment should be immediately available in the event of a paediatric cardiac arrest. Suggestions have also been made regarding the storage, checking and maintenance of this equipment. Aids to calculating drug doses and equipment sizes for paediatric resuscitation have also been outlined.

Chapter 3

Recognition of respiratory failure and circulatory shock

Introduction

The prompt recognition and treatment of potential respiratory failure and shock in children are essential if the dire situation of cardiopulmonary arrest and its associated poor prognosis is to be avoided (Zaritsky *et al.*, 1987; ALSG, 2001).

The aim of this chapter is to understand the principles of the recognition of respiratory failure and circulatory shock.

Objectives

At the end of the chapter the reader will be able to:

- define respiratory failure and circulatory shock
- discuss why early recognition of potential respiratory failure and shock is important
- describe a rapid assessment of respiratory function
- describe a rapid assessment of cardiovascular function
- describe a rapid assessment of neurological function
- describe a rapid assessment of the child's general appearance.

Definitions of respiratory failure and circulatory shock

- *Respiratory failure* is a clinical state characterized by inadequate ventilation or oxygenation. A compensated state may precede respiratory failure: the child may be able to maintain adequate ventilation by increasing the respiratory rate or depth; this will be evident by the presence of increased work in breathing and tachycardia (American Academy of Pediatrics, 1997).
- *Circulatory shock* is a clinical state characterized by inadequate delivery of oxygen and metabolic substances to meet the needs of the tissues. It can be classified as compensated shock (normal blood pressure) or decompensated shock (low blood pressure) (American Academy of Pediatrics, 1997).

Importance of rapid recognition of potential respiratory failure and circulatory shock

Cardiopulmonary arrests in children are rarely sudden events and are rarely caused by a primary cardiac pathology (ALSG, 2001). They generally

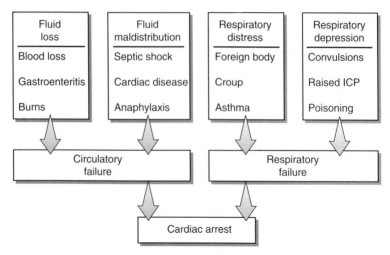

Fig. 3.1 Pathways leading to cardiac arrest in infants and children (reproduced from ALSG, 2001, with kind permission).

follow a period of profound hypoxia associated with respiratory failure and/or shock (Fig. 3.1). As a result, by the time the child has deteriorated into a state of cardiopulmonary arrest, all the organs of the body will have suffered from the effects of hypoxia and ischaemia (Lucking *et al.*, 1986).

Consequently, organs particularly sensitive to hypoxia and anoxia, e.g. the brain and kidneys, are often seriously damaged by the time cardiopulmonary arrest occurs. In these situations, although CPR may restore a cardiac output, the child often then either dies in the ensuing days from multisystem failure or survives with neurological damage (Zideman, 1994). It is therefore essential to try to prevent deterioration to cardiopulmonary arrest by rapidly recognizing and treating respiratory and/or circulatory insufficiencies.

Rapid assessment of respiratory function

The rapid assessment of respiratory function involves the evaluation of:

- work of breathing
- effectiveness of breathing
- adequacy of ventilation.

Work of breathing

Healthy spontaneous breathing is quiet and is accomplished with minimal effort. An increased respiratory rate, chest recession, noisy respirations, accessory muscle use and nasal flaring are signs of an increased work of breathing.

Table 3.1 Normal respiratory rates by age at rest (reproduced from ALSG, 2001, with kind permission)

Age (years)	Respiratory rate (breaths per minute)
<1	30–40
1–2	25–35
2–5	25–30
5–12	20–25
>12	15–20

Respiratory rate

- Normal respiratory rates are detailed in Table 3.1.
- Tachypnoea at rest can be caused by airway disease, lung disease or metabolic acidosis.
- Tachypnoea is usually one of the first indications of respiratory distress.
- Slow or irregular respirations in acutely ill infants and children are an ominous sign. Possible causes include fatigue, hypothermia and CNS depression. A slow respiratory rate in an exhausted child is a sign of deterioration, rather than improvement, and is a pre-terminal sign.
- A trend of respiratory rates can be very useful and is sometimes more accurate than the first recorded rate (American Academy of Pediatrics, 2000).

Chest recession

- Intercostal, subcostal or sternal recession are signs of increased work of breathing.
- It is particularly visible in infants (Fig. 3.2) because their chest walls are more compliant – the chest wall is less muscular and thinner and the inward excursion of the skin and soft tissue between the ribs is more visible (American Academy of Pediatrics, 2000).
- If seen in older children (i.e. over 6 years of age), it is probably indicative of serious respiratory difficulties.
- The degree of recession correlates with severity of respiratory distress.

Noisy respirations

- **Stridor** – an inspiratory, high-pitched sound indicating partial upper airway obstruction; causes include, e.g. croup, foreign body aspiration, infection and oedema (American Academy of Pediatrics, 2000).
- **Wheeze** – whistling sound more pronounced on expiration, indicating narrowing of the lower airways; the two most common causes are asthma (generally in children >1 year old) and bronchiolitis (generally in infants <1 year old) (ALSG, 2001).
- **Grunting** – short low-pitched sound resulting from exhalation against a partially closed glottis; it is an attempt to keep the alveoli open for gas exchange (and prevent airway collapse at the end of expiration)

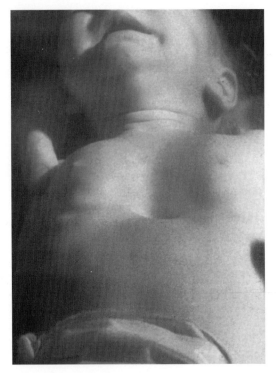

Fig. 3.2   Chest recession (reproduced with kind permission from the Advanced Life Support Group, Manchester, UK).

(American Academy of Pediatrics, 2000). It is a sign of serious respiratory distress and is characteristically observed in infants (ALSG, 2001).

Accessory muscle use
Use of the sternomastoid muscle may result in bobbing of the head up and down with each breath – on inhalation the neck is extended and on exhalation the head falls forward resulting in the characteristic 'head bobbing' effect.

Nasal flaring
Nasal flaring (exaggerated opening of the nostrils) is commonly seen in infants with respiratory distress.

Child position
- Sniffing position – the child is making an attempt to line up the axes of the airways to open the airway and maximize airflow (American Academy of Pediatrics, 2000).
- Tripod position – leaning forward on outstretched arms in an attempt to use accessory muscles.

> NB: Children with a depressed cerebral function, e.g. due to poisoning or a raised intracranial pressure, may present with respiratory inadequacy without the signs of increased work of breathing. This is due to a depressed respiratory drive.

Effectiveness of breathing

The effectiveness of breathing can be assessed by:

- chest movement
- air entry/tidal volume (a silent chest is an ominous sign); look, listen and feel and auscultate over the midaxillary lines
- oxygen saturation monitoring or pulse oximetry – a useful non-invasive method of assessing oxygen saturation (it does not give an indication of the effectiveness of ventilation); saturation levels < 90% on air and < 95% on high-flow oxygen are considered low (ALSG, 2001); always interpret oxygen saturation level together with work of breathing, because a child in respiratory distress or in the early stages of respiratory failure may be able to maintain 'adequate' oxygen levels by increasing the work of breathing and respiratory rate (American Academy of Pediatrics, 2000).

Signs of inadequate ventilation

The assessment of heart rate, skin colour and mental status can help the nurse to determine whether ventilation is adequate:

Heart rate
- Initially tachycardia in the older infant and child (a non-specific sign).
- Severe hypoxia leads to bradycardia (a pre-terminal sign).

Skin colour
- Initially pallor. Hypoxia will lead to catecholamine release, causing vasoconstriction.
- Central cyanosis is a late and pre-terminal sign of hypoxia.
- NB: If the child is anaemic, cyanosis may not be present even when hypoxia is severe.
- NB: Cyanosis may be 'normal' if the child has congenital heart disease.
- In dark-skinned children, the lips and mucous membranes may be the best places to observe skin colour (American Academy of Pediatrics, 2000).

Mental status
Hypoxia will affect the mental status of the child. Initially the child may be agitated, drowsy, or may fail to recognize/acknowledge his or her parents. If uncorrected, this may lead to unconsciousness and generalized muscular hypotonia (floppy child). A useful method of rapidly assessing the mental status is by using the AVPU scale:

- **A**lert
- Responds to **V**oice

- Responds to **P**ainful stimuli
- **U**nconscious.

AVPU categorizes motor response, based on simple responses to stimuli (American Academy of Pediatrics, 2000).

Rapid assessment of cardiovascular function

Assessment of the cardiovascular function includes evaluation of:

- heart rate
- pulse volume
- capillary refill
- skin temperature
- blood pressure
- respiratory system
- urine output
- mental status.

Heart rate
- Normal heart rates are shown in Table 3.2.
- Tachycardia is a non-specific sign (there are numerous causes of tachycardia including anxiety, excitement, pyrexia and pain).
- Initially there is an increase in heart rate (caused by release of catecholamines to compensate for the decreased stroke volume).
- Bradycardia is an ominous sign.
- A trend of increasing or decreasing heart rate recordings may be useful, suggesting worsening hypoxia or shock or improvement following effective treatment (American Academy of Pediatrics, 2000).

Pulse volume
Absent peripheral pulses and weak central pulses indicate poor cardiac output and are signs of advanced stages of shock.

Capillary refill
Capillary refill longer than 2 seconds may indicate poor skin perfusion.
 Capillary refill can be estimated by elevating a limb above the level of the heart (ensures assessment of arteriolar capillary refill and not venous

Table 3.2   Normal range of heart rates by age (reproduced from ALSG, 2001, with kind permission)

Age (years)	Heart rate (beats per minute)
<1	110–160
1–2	100–150
2–5	95–140
5–12	80–120
>12	60–100

stasis) and blanching the skin for 5 seconds (Fig. 3.3). The normal capillary refill time is up to 2 seconds and the ambient temperature must be warm.

Skin temperature
- If perfusion is adequate, the child's skin near the wrists and ankles should be warm (American Academy of Pediatrics, 2000).
- When cardiac output decreases, cooling of the skin starts peripherally and extends proximally towards the trunk (Joly and Weil, 1969).
- As shock worsens, a line of coldness can be identified moving centrally.
- NB: If the child is cold, core perfusion may be normal despite 'abnormal' skin perfusion owing to peripheral shutdown.

Blood pressure
- Not a very useful sign – a child can be in shock and still have a normal blood pressure (compensated shock).
- NB: Hypotension is a late sign of shock (decompensated shock) and cardiac arrest may be imminent.
- Minimum systolic blood pressure readings are displayed in Table 3.3.

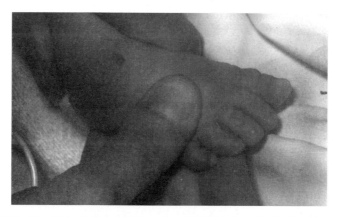

Fig. 3.3   Checking capillary refill (reproduced with kind permission from the Advanced Life Support Group, Manchester, UK).

Table 3.3   Systolic blood pressure by age (reproduced from ALSG, 2001, with kind permission)

Age (years)	Systolic blood pressure (mmHg)
< 1	70–90
1–2	80–95
2–5	80–100
5–12	90–110
> 12	100–120

- For children > 1 year, a suggested simple formula to ascertain the minimum acceptable systolic blood pressure is 70 + 2 × child's age in years (American Academy of Pediatrics, 2000).

Respiratory system
Metabolic acidosis resulting from circulatory failure will cause a tachypnoea and an increased tidal volume (without chest recession).

Urine output
Poor urine output (<1 ml/kg/hour in children and <2 ml/kg/hour in infants) indicates inadequate renal perfusion.

Mental status
Poor cerebral perfusion will often cause agitation initially, followed by drowsiness and then unconsciousness if not corrected.

Rapid assessment of neurological function

A rapid assessment of neurological function involves evaluating conscious level, posture and pupils:

- *Conscious level.* Use the AVPU scale (see above); applying pressure to the sternum or pulling frontal hair are two acceptable methods of delivering the painful central stimulus (ALSG, 2001); a child who only responds to pain has a significant degree of coma corresponding to 8 or less on the Glasgow Coma Scale (ALSG, 2001).
- *Posture.* Decorticate posturing (flexed arms, extended legs) or decerebrate posturing (extended arms, extended legs) are signs of serious neurological dysfunction (ALSG, 2001).
- *Pupils.* Causes of an abnormal pupillary response include drugs, hypoxia, convulsions and impending brain stem herniation (American Academy of Pediatrics, 2000); dilatation, unreactivity or inequality indicate possible serious cerebral disorder (ALSG, 2001).

Neurological function can be adversely affected by both respiratory and cardiovascular dysfunction. In addition, neurological dysfunction can adversely affect both of these systems.

Rapid assessment of the child's general appearance

A rapid assessment of the child's general appearance is important when ascertaining how severe the illness or injury is, the need for treatment and the response to therapy (American Academy of Pediatrics, 2000). The child's general appearance provides an indication of the adequacy of ventilation, oxygenation, tissue perfusion, cerebral perfusion and neurological function.

The so-called 'tickles' (TICLS) mnemonic (American Academy of Pediatrics, 2000) can help with the assessment of the child's general appearance:

- Tone. Good muscle tone or limp, listless or flaccid? Is the child vigorous and resisting examination?
- Interactiveness. How alert is the child? Attentive and easily distracted? Reaching for, grasping and playing with a toy? Uninterested in playing or interacting?
- Consolability. Consoled or comforted by the carer? Crying and agitation unrelieved by gentle reassurance?
- Look/gaze. Good eye contact? 'Nobody home', glassy-eyed stare?
- Speech/cry. Speech or cry, strong and spontaneous, or weak, muffled or hoarse?

NB: **An alert, interactive child may still be critically ill, e.g. in a toxicological or trauma emergency.**

Summary

A systematic approach to the rapid assessment of seriously ill children has been described. This rapid assessment of the respiratory, cardiovascular and neurological functions, together with an assessment of the child's general appearance, can help to ascertain whether the child is seriously ill or not. The prompt recognition and treatment of potential respiratory failure and shock in children are essential if the dire situation of cardiopulmonary arrest and its associated poor prognosis is to be avoided.

Chapter 4

Basic life support

Introduction

The aetiology of cardiopulmonary arrests in infants and children differs from that in adults (Hazinski, 1995). They are normally secondary to either respiratory or circulatory failure, and rarely result from a primary cardiac event. Respiratory failure is the most common cause.

The priorities and sequence of paediatric basic life support (BLS) therefore follow the principle that 'early effective oxygenation and ventilation must be established as quickly as possible' (European Resuscitation Council, 1998). Indeed survival from cardiopulmonary arrest is dependent mainly upon the immediate provision of effective rescue ventilation (Friesen *et al.*, 1982).

BLS refers to maintaining an open airway and supporting breathing and circulation without the use of equipment other than a protective shield (Handley, 1999). In the hospital setting the availability of additional personnel and equipment (particularly airway/ventilation adjuncts) makes it necessary to adapt the conventional BLS guidelines. However, health-care professionals must still have a working knowledge of BLS in case they need to perform it outside their normal working environment.

The aim of this chapter is to understand the principles of the European Resuscitation Council BLS guidelines.

Objectives

At the end of the chapter the reader will be able to:

- outline potential hazards when attempting BLS
- discuss the initial assessment and sequence of actions in BLS
- outline the principles of basic airway management
- describe two methods of ventilation
- describe the correct procedure for chest compressions
- describe the recovery position
- outline the management of foreign body airway obstruction
- outline the principles of safer handling during CPR.

Potential hazards when attempting BLS

It is important to eliminate or at least minimize any potential hazards associated with attempting BLS (Resuscitation Council (UK), 2000a). Potential hazards could include the environment, infection and poisoning.

In addition, national guidelines for safer handling during CPR should be followed (Resuscitation Council (UK), 2001).

Environment

Although unlikely to be a problem in the hospital setting, environmental hazards to resuscitation could include traffic, electricity, gas, etc.

Infection

There have only been 15 documented cases of the transmission of infection through mouth-to-mouth ventilation, none of which involved HIV or hepatitis B virus (Mejicano and Maki, 1998). Although there is a theoretical risk of infectious disease transmission while performing BLS, the risk is very low (Mejicano and Maki, 1998).

However the re-emergence of tuberculosis is a cause for concern, particularly as it can be transmitted through mouth-to-mouth ventilation (Haley *et al.*, 1989).

Most out-of-hospital paediatric arrests occur at home and surveys of family members have demonstrated that infection risk is not a concern when resuscitating a loved one (Dracup *et al.*, 1998). However, both healthcare workers and laypersons are often reluctant to perform mouth-to-mouth ventilation, most commonly because of a fear of contracting HIV (Brenner *et al.*, 1996). Consequently, there are a variety of barrier devices available (Fig. 4.1); facemasks with one-way valves prevent the transmission of bacteria, while face shields are less effective (Centers for Disease Control, 1991).

Blood is the single most important source of the transmission of HIV and hepatitis B virus. There is therefore a theoretical risk of their transmission during mouth-to-mouth ventilation in cases of facial trauma, or if there are breaks in the skin around the lips or soft tissues of the oral cavity mucosa (Piazza *et al.*, 1989). Caution is particularly warranted in these situations.

Universal precautions should apply to blood and cerebrospinal, synovial, pleural, peritoneal, pericardial and amniotic fluids and any body fluid containing visible blood (Centers for Disease Control, 1988). Care with sharps is paramount as both HIV and the hepatitis B virus have been contracted by healthcare workers following needle-stick injuries (Marcus, 1988).

Poisoning

The child's exhaled air should be avoided in hydrogen cyanide or hydrogen sulphide gas poisoning. Ventilation should be undertaken using a non-return-valve system.

Corrosive chemicals, e.g. strong acids, alkalis or paraquat, can easily be absorbed through the skin and respiratory tract; care should be taken when handling the child's clothes and bodily fluids, particularly vomit (Resuscitation Council (UK), 2000a). Protective clothing and gloves should be worn.

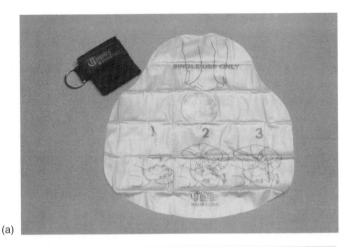

(a)

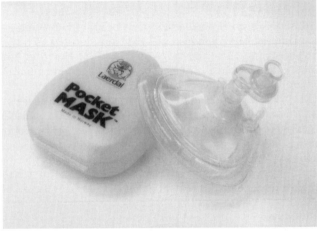

(b)

Fig. 4.1   Barrier devices: (a) a face shield (Timesco of London); (b) a pocket mask (Laerdal).

Initial assessment and sequence of actions in BLS

The initial assessment and sequence of actions in BLS outside the health-care environment are outlined below, based on the European Resuscitation Council paediatric BLS 2001 (Fig. 4.2). Infant and child are defined by age, as follows:

• Infant < 1 year
• Child 1–8 years (use common sense).

The traditional 'ABC' sequence remains pertinent. On finding a collapsed, apparently lifeless infant/child, ensure it is safe to approach and then check responsiveness.

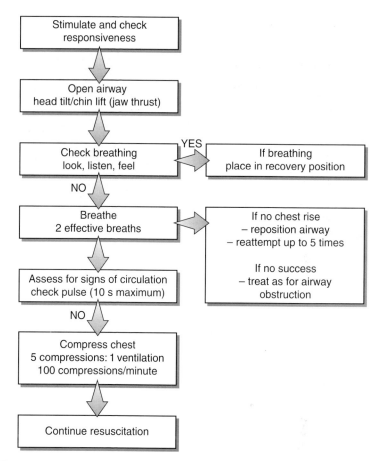

Fig. 4.2 European Resuscitation Council paediatric basic life support algorithm 2001 (with permission of Aurum Pharmaceuticals).

Check responsiveness

Infant   Gently rub the chest, blow on the face, tickle the feet.

Child   Gently shake the shoulders (careful if cervical spinal injury suspected) and ask loudly 'are you all right?'.

Response   Leave the infant/child in the position in which he has been found, provided there is no further danger. Establish the likely cause of the collapse and get help if necessary.

No response   Call out for help and proceed to assessing the airway. If there is no history of trauma, it may be worth moving an infant/small child near to a phone so that the emergency services can be quickly alerted.

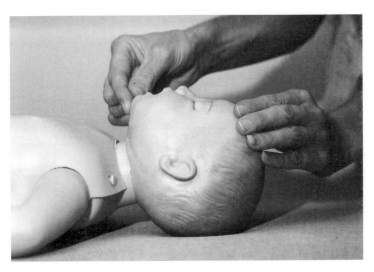

Fig. 4.3   Head tilt/chin lift manoeuvre.

Open airway

Turn the infant/child onto his back (unless full assessment is possible in the position in which he has been found). Open the airway by tilting the head and lifting the chin (Fig. 4.3) (Roth *et al.*, 1998) (caution if cervical spine injury suspected). Look in the mouth and remove any obvious obstruction and then check breathing.

Check breathing

While maintaining an open airway check for signs of breathing (Fig. 4.4) (more than an occasional gasp or weak attempts at breathing) for up to 10 seconds:

- Look for rise and fall of the chest and abdomen.
- Listen for airflow at the mouth and nose.
- Feel for airflow on your cheek.

It can sometimes be difficult to establish whether the infant/child is breathing (Ruppert *et al.*, 1999) and it is important to differentiate ineffective, gasping or obstructed respirations from effective respirations (Noc *et al.*, 1994; Poets *et al.*, 1999). If uncertain whether the infant/child is breathing deliver rescue breaths.

Infant/child breathing   Place in the recovery position (caution if history of trauma), check for continued breathing and ensure help is on the way.

Infant/child not breathing   Send someone else for help and deliver rescue breaths.

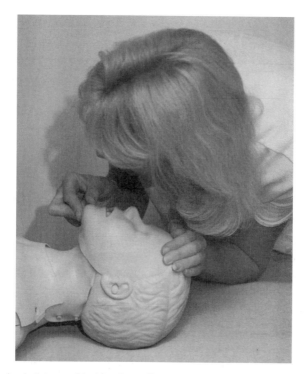

Fig. 4.4 Look, listen and feel for signs of breathing.

Breathe

Deliver two effective breaths. Allow up to five attempts to achieve this and then proceed to assess signs of circulation.

Assess signs of circulation

Allow up to 10 seconds to assess for signs of circulation: look, listen and feel for signs of breathing, coughing or movement of the casualty. Also check for the pulse for no longer than 10 seconds:

Infant Check for the brachial pulse (Fig. 4.5) – short, chubby necks in infants make checking for the carotid pulse difficult (Cavallaro and Melker, 1983). The brachial pulse is located on the inside of the infant's upper arm, in between the elbow and the shoulder.

Child Check for the carotid pulse (Mather and O'Kelly, 1996) – locate the thyroid cartilage (Adam's apple) with two or three fingers from one hand (maintain head tilt with the other), then slide the fingers into the groove in between the trachea and sternocleidomastoid muscles and then gently palpate.

Only check the pulse if trained to do so, as it can be difficult to reliably determine its presence or absence (Flesche *et al.*, 1994; Eberle *et al.*, 1996;

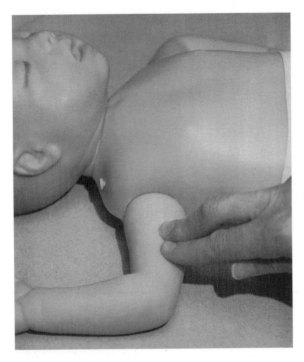

Fig. 4.5   Check for brachial pulse.

Bahr *et al.*, 1997). Teaching laypersons how to check for the pulse is not recommended. Instead they should be taught to look for signs of circulation in response to rescue breaths (American Heart Association, 2000).

Signs of circulation present   Continue rescue breaths at a rate of 20 per minute and check for signs of circulation every minute.

No signs of circulation or unsure   Compress the chest at a rate of 100 per minute combining compressions with rescue breaths at a ratio of 5 : 1 (five compressions to one rescue breath).

When to get help
More than one rescuer   One starts CPR while the other gets help.

Lone rescuer   Perform CPR for 1 minute before getting help (it may be possible to carry an infant/small child and perform CPR/get help simultaneously).

Principles of basic airway management
The airway in an unconscious child can easily become obstructed by a combination of flexion of the neck, relaxation of the jaw, displacement of

the tongue against the posterior wall of the pharynx and collapse of the hypopharynx (Hudgel and Hendricks, 1988; Abernethy *et al.*, 1990). In some cases just opening the airway may revive the child.

The airway can be opened by tilting the head and lifting the chin. This will help to open the airway and bring the tongue forward from the posterior wall of the pharynx (the tongue is the most common cause of airway obstruction in an unconscious child (Ruben *et al.*, 1961)). The neutral position in an infant and the 'sniffing the morning air' position in a child are recommended (ALSG, 2001).

Care should be taken not to press on the soft tissues under the chin as this may obstruct the airway. Blind finger sweeps are not recommended (European Resuscitation Council, 1998). Although cervical spine injuries are rare in infants and children (American Heart Association, 2000), if there is a history of trauma, the jaw thrust rather than head tilt/chin lift is recommended (ALSG, 2001) (see pp. 50–51).

Principles of mouth-to-mouth ventilation

Mouth-to-mouth ventilation is a quick, effective way to provide adequate oxygenation and ventilation in a casualty who is not breathing (Wenzel *et al.*, 1994).

However, particular attention to the correct technique is essential. The most common cause of failure to ventilate is improper positioning of the head and chin (Idris *et al.*, 1996).

Mouth-to-mouth-and-nose ventilation (infant)

1. Position the infant in a supine position (preferably on a table or similar).
2. Place the infant's head in a neutral position and maintain head tilt and chin lift.
3. If trained to do so, apply a face shield barrier device.
4. Take a deep breath in.
5. Bend forwards from the hips leaning down towards the infant's nose and mouth.
6. Place your lips around the infant's lips and nose, and ensure an airtight seal.
7. Breathe out steadily into the infant's mouth and nose over 1–1½ seconds and observe for chest rise (Zideman and Spearpoint, 1999). The correct breath volume is one that causes the chest to rise, without causing excessive gastric distension (Berg *et al.*, 1998).
8. While still maintaining head tilt and chin lift, remove your mouth and watch for chest fall, as the air comes out.
9. Take another breath in (pausing to take a breath will maximize the oxygen content and minimize the carbon dioxide content in the delivered breaths (Tendrup *et al.*, 1989)) and repeat steps 5–9.
10. Perform up to five breaths to achieve two effective breaths.

11. If the rescuer has a small mouth it may not be possible to cover both the infant's nose and mouth (Dembofsky *et al.*, 1999). In this situation, mouth-to-nose ventilation may be adequate (Tonkin *et al.*, 1995).

Mouth-to-mouth ventilation (child)

1. Position the child in a supine position (a smaller child preferably on a table or similar).
2. Kneel in a comfortable position with the knees a shoulder width apart, at the side of the child at the level of his nose and mouth.
3. Rest back to sit on the heels in the low kneeling position.
4. Place the child's head in a 'sniffing the morning air' position and maintain head tilt and chin lift.
5. If trained to do so, apply a face shield barrier device.
6. Pinch the soft part of the child's nose.
7. Take a deep breath in.
8. Bend forwards from the hips leaning down towards the child's nose and mouth.
9. Place your lips around the child's lips and ensure an airtight seal.
10. Breathe out steadily into the child's mouth over 1–1½ seconds and observe for chest rise (Zideman and Spearpoint, 1999). The correct breath volume is one that causes the chest to rise, without causing excessive gastric distension (Berg *et al.*, 1998).
11. While still maintaining head tilt and chin lift, remove your mouth and watch for chest fall, as the air comes out.
12. Take another breath (pausing to take a breath will maximize the oxygen content and minimize the carbon dioxide content in the delivered breaths (Tendrup *et al.*, 1989)) and repeat steps 8–11.
13. Perform up to five breaths to achieve two effective breaths.

Ineffective delivery of breaths

If it is difficult to deliver effective breaths:

- ensure adequate head tilt and chin lift
- reposition the airway (slight readjustment may be all that is required)
- recheck the child's mouth and remove any obstruction
- ensure an airtight seal
- ensure the casualty's nose is pinched during ventilation
- allow up to five attempts to achieve two effective breaths – if unsuccessful proceed to the management of choking guidelines (see below).

Complications of gastric inflation

Gastric inflation is commonly associated with mouth-to-mouth ventilation (Idris *et al.*, 1995), particularly if the rescue breaths are performed rapidly (Melker, 1985). It occurs when the pressure in the oesophagus exceeds the opening pressure of the lower oesophageal sphincter, resulting in the sphincter opening (Basket *et al.*, 1996). During CPR the oesophageal sphincter relaxes, thus increasing the likelihood of gastric inflation (Bowman *et al.*, 1995).

Complications of gastric inflation include:

- regurgitation (Stone *et al.*, 1998)
- aspiration (Lawes and Baskett, 1987)
- pneumonia (Bjork *et al.*, 1982)
- diaphragm elevation, restricted lung movements and reduced lung compliance (Berg *et al.*, 1998).

Gastric inflation can be minimized if rescue breaths are delivered slowly (over 1–1½ seconds). Cricoid pressure, described on pages 53–54, can also help.

Principles of chest compressions

Mechanisms of blood flow

Chest compressions create blood flow by increasing intrathoracic pressure or directly compressing the heart (Maier *et al.*, 1984). Even if chest compressions are being performed correctly, cardiac output is still only about 30% of normal, with systolic blood pressures of between 60 and 80 mmHg being achieved (Paradis *et al.*, 1989). During chest compressions, blood flow can be maximized by positioning the patient horizontal, and using the recommended chest compression force, duration, rate and ratio.

Chest compressions in an infant

Location Lower half of the sternum (Orlowski, 1984; Phillips and Zideman, 1986) – two fingers on the sternum, one finger's breadth below the nipple line (Fig. 4.6); a more effective technique is the thumb technique, with the hands encircling the chest (Fig. 4.7) (David, 1988) – this is the preferred method when two healthcare professionals are present (American Heart Association, 2000). (Compression of the xiphoid process should be avoided as this may injure the liver, stomach or spleen (Thaler and Krause, 1962).)

Depth One-third to one-half of the depth of the chest.

Rate 100 per minute, coordinated with ventilations.

Ratio 5 compressions : 1 ventilation.

Chest compressions in a child

Location Heel of one hand on the sternum, two fingers' breadth above the ziphisternum (Fig. 4.8).

Depth One-third to one-half of the depth of the chest.

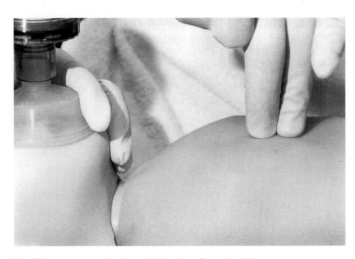

Fig. 4.6 Chest compression in an infant: two-finger technique.

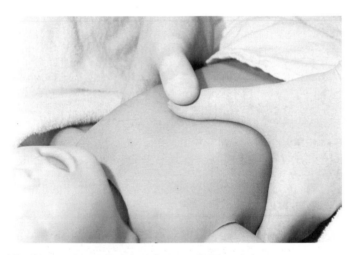

Fig. 4.7 Chest compression in an infant: two-thumb technique.

Rate 100 per minute.

Ratio 5 compressions : 1 ventilation.

Chest compressions in an older child

In children over approximately 8 years of age it may be necessary to adopt the 'adult' two-handed technique for chest compressions (Fig. 4.9), in order to achieve effective chest compressions (Resuscitation Council (UK), 2000c).

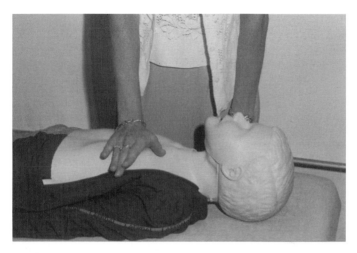

Fig. 4.8   Chest compression in a child.

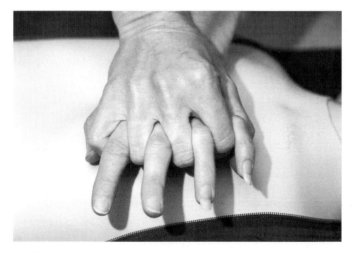

Fig. 4.9   Chest compression in an older child.

Location   Heel of one hand on the lower half of the sternum, with the other hand on top.

Depth   One-third to one-half of the depth of the chest.

Rate   100 per minute.

Ratio   15 compressions : 2 ventilations.

Duration

Cerebral and coronary perfusion is optimum when 50% of the cycle is devoted to the chest compression phase and 50% to the chest relaxation phase (Handley and Handley, 1995).

Rate

A chest compression rate of 100 per minute is required to achieve optimum blood flow during CPR. The rate refers to the speed of compressions rather than the actual number delivered per minute (Resuscitation Council (UK), 2000c).

When chest compressions are interrupted to provide ventilations, the actual number delivered will therefore be < 100 per minute and will vary from rescuer to rescuer depending upon the time taken to position the head, open the airway and deliver the rescue breaths (Whyte and Wyllie, 1999).

(Once the patient has been intubated and chest compressions and ventilations are asynchronous, the number of compressions delivered will then be approximately 100 per minute.)

Recovery position

Although there are a number of recovery positions currently advocated, no single one can be endorsed. However, the position adopted should:

• be stable
• maintain a patent airway
• maintain a stable cervical spine
• avoid application of pressure on the chest that restricts breathing
• minimize the risk of aspiration
• limit pressure on bony prominences and peripheral nerves
• enable visualization of the child's breathing and colour
• allow access to the child for interventions
• be easy and safe to achieve (including repositioning if required).

Management of foreign body airway obstruction

Complete obstruction of the airway by a foreign body is a life-threatening emergency and is often characterized by a sudden inability to talk, maximal respiratory effort, development of cyanosis and clutching of the neck.

In partial airway obstruction, the child will be distressed, may cough and may have a wheeze. In complete airway obstruction, the child will be unable to speak, breathe or cough and will eventually go unconscious.

Treatment of a choking infant

If the infant is choking, but able to breathe, encourage him to cough. If the infant is choking but either is unable to breathe or is breathing but shows

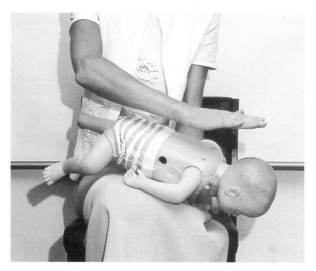

Fig. 4.10   Management of foreign body aspiration in an infant: back slaps.

signs of becoming weak or stops breathing or coughing:

1. Remove any obvious foreign body from the mouth, but do not perform blind finger sweeps as these may further impact the foreign body and may cause pharyngeal trauma (Hartrey and Bingham, 1995; Kabbani and Goodwin, 1995).
2. Position the infant in a prone position resting on your forearm, with the head lower than the chest and the airway open. Ensure the head is well supported.
3. Deliver up to five sharp slaps (Fig. 4.10) between the scapulae using the heel of the hand. If the back slaps fail to dislodge the foreign body, proceed to chest thrusts.
4. Turn the infant into a supine position, with the head lower than the chest and the airway open.
5. Deliver up to five chest thrusts to the sternum (Fig. 4.11) (similar to chest compressions, but more vigorous, sharper and slower, at a rate of one every second).
6. Recheck the mouth and carefully remove any visible foreign body.
7. Reposition the airway using the head tilt/chin lift procedure.
8. Reassess breathing. If the infant is breathing, place in a lateral position and monitor. If the infant is not breathing, attempt rescue breaths (up to five attempts to achieve two effective breaths).
9. If the airway remains obstructed, repeat steps 2–8 as appropriate.

NB: Abdominal thrusts are not recommended in infants (Resuscitation Council (UK), 2000c).

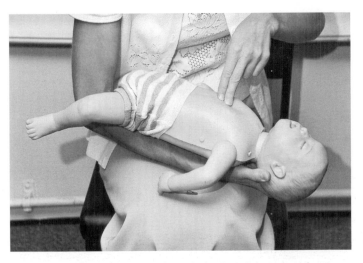

Fig. 4.11   Management of foreign body aspiration in an infant: chest thrusts.

Treatment of a choking child

If the child is choking, but able to breathe, encourage him to cough. If the child is choking but either is unable to breathe or is breathing but shows signs of becoming weak or stops breathing or coughing:

1. Remove any obvious foreign body from the mouth, but do not perform blind finger sweeps as these may further impact the foreign body (Zideman and Spearpoint, 1999) and may cause pharyngeal trauma (Hartrey and Bingham, 1995; Kabbani and Goodwin, 1995).
2. Position the child in a prone position, with the head lower than the chest and the airway open.
3. Deliver up to five sharp slaps between the scapulae (Fig. 4.12) using the heel of the hand. If the back slaps fail to dislodge the foreign body, proceed to chest thrusts.
4. Turn the child into a supine position, with the head lower than the chest and the airway open.
5. Deliver up to five chest thrusts to the sternum (similar to chest compressions, but more vigorous, sharper and slower, at a rate of one every 3 seconds).
6. Recheck the mouth and carefully remove any visible foreign body.
7. Reposition the airway using the head tilt/chin lift procedure.
8. Reassess breathing. If the child is breathing, place in a lateral position and monitor. If the child is not breathing, attempt rescue breaths (up to five attempts to achieve two effective breaths).
9. If the airway remains obstructed, deliver up to five further back slaps (steps 2–3). If these are ineffective, proceed to abdominal thrusts.

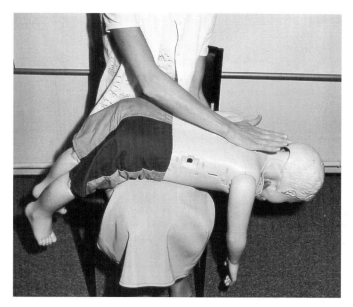

Fig. 4.12   Management of foreign body aspiration in a child: back slaps.

10. Deliver up to five abdominal thrusts (see below).
11. Repeat steps 6–8 as appropriate and restart cycle with back slaps if necessary.
12. Alternate between chest thrusts and abdominal thrusts in subsequent cycles.

Abdominal thrusts in a conscious child

1. Stand or kneel behind the child.
2. Position your arms directly underneath the child's axillae and encircle the torso.
3. Bend the child forward.
4. Place the thumb side of one fist against the child's abdomen, in the midline just above the umbilicus but well below the xiphoid process.
5. Grasp the fist with the other hand.
6. Exert up to five quick inward and upward thrusts. Avoid touching the xiphoid process and lower margins of the rib cage because any force applied to these structures could damage internal organs (Cowan *et al.*, 1987; Bintz and Cogbill, 1996; Majumdar and Sedman, 1998).

(American Academy of Pediatrics, 1997)

Abdominal thrusts in an unconscious child

1. Place the child in a supine position.
2. Straddle the child's hips or kneel at the side.

3. Place the heel of one hand on the child's abdomen, in the midline just above the umbilicus but well below the xiphoid process.
4. Position the other hand on top of the first.
5. Exert up to five quick inward and upward thrusts. Avoid touching the xiphoid process and lower margins of the rib cage because any force applied to these structures could damage internal organs (Cowan *et al.*, 1987; Bintz and Cogbill, 1996; Majumdar and Sedman, 1998).

(American Academy of Pediatrics, 1997)

> If teaching a layperson the management of foreign body airway obstruction, it is recommended to advise that CPR should be undertaken for 1 minute and then the emergency services activated if a choking infant or child loses consciousness (American Heart Association, 2000). This is because chest compressions could generate sufficient pressure to remove a foreign body (Langelle *et al.*, 2000).

Principles of safer handling during CPR

The Resuscitation Council (UK), in their publication 'Guidance for Safer Handling during Resuscitation in Hospitals' (2001), has issued guidelines concerning safer handling during CPR. Although they are mainly aimed at the resuscitation of adults, some are applicable to paediatric resuscitation. A brief overview of these guidelines is given below.

Environmental hazards Remove any hazards, ensure that the bed (resuscitaire) brakes are on and lower cotsides if they are up.

Ventilation and intubation Move the bed away from the wall and remove the backrest to allow access; stand at the top of the bed facing the child with the feet in a walk/stand position and avoid prolonged static postures.

Chest compressions Ensure the bed is at a height which places the child between the knee and mid-thigh of the practitioner performing chest compressions. Stand at the side of the bed with the feet shoulder-width apart, position the shoulders directly over the child's sternum and, keeping the arms straight, compress the chest, ensuring that the force for compressions results from flexing the hips. Chest compressions can also be performed by kneeling with both knees on the bed.

CPR on a fixed-height bed, couch or trolley If necessary, stand on steps or a firm stool, with a non-slip surface and which is wide enough to permit the practitioner's feet to be shoulder-width apart; do not kneel on a couch or trolley.

Summary

The initial assessment and sequence of actions in BLS in infants and children have been discussed. The principles of basic airway management, ventilation and chest compressions have been described. The management of foreign body airway obstruction has been outlined. As respiratory failure is the most common cause of cardiac arrest in childhood, particular attention to securing the airway and providing adequate ventilation is paramount.

Chapter 5

Airway management and ventilation

Introduction

The priorities and sequence of paediatric basic life support (BLS) follow the principle that 'early effective oxygenation and ventilation must be established as quickly as possible' (ERC, 1998). Indeed survival from cardio-pulmonary arrest is mainly dependent upon the immediate provision of effective rescue ventilations (Friesen *et al.*, 1982). Effective airway management and ventilation during CPR are therefore paramount.

The aim of this chapter is to understand the principles of airway management and ventilation.

Objectives

At the end of the chapter the reader will be able to:

- discuss relevant anatomy and physiology
- list the causes of airway obstruction
- outline the recognition of airway obstruction
- describe simple techniques to open and clear the airway
- discuss the procedure for the application of cricoid pressure
- discuss the use of oropharyngeal and nasopharyngeal airways
- outline the role of the laryngeal mask airway
- describe the procedure for tracheal intubation
- describe two methods of ventilation.

Relevant anatomy and physiology

Anatomy and physiology related to airway management and ventilation in infants and children include:

- A large head, short neck tends to cause flexion of the neck.
- The face and mandible are small.
- Orthodontic appliances may be loose.
- The tongue is relatively large – in an unconscious child it often obstructs the airway and can also impede visualization during tracheal intubation.
- The floor of the mouth is easily compressible – care should therefore be taken when positioning the fingers during airway manoeuvres.

- The epiglottis is horse-shoe shaped and projects posteriorly at 45 degrees – this makes tracheal intubation more difficult to perform (in infants a straight blade laryngoscope is preferred).
- The larynx is high and anterior.
- The larynx is funnel shaped with the cricoid cartilage being the narrowest part of the upper airway (compared to the larynx in adults).
- The cricoid cartilage is particularly susceptible to oedema – because the cuff of a tracheal tube tends to lie at this level, uncuffed tubes are preferred in children pre-puberty.
- The trachea is short and soft – it can easily be compressed if the neck is over-extended.
- Tracheal tube displacement is more likely because the trachea is short.
- Upper and lower airways are relatively small – they can easily become obstructed. Even a small reduction in airway size can lead to a significant increase in airflow resistance and work of breathing, particularly if the airflow is turbulent, e.g. during crying (Cote and Todres, 1990) – hence children with airway obstruction should be kept as calm and quiet as possible (American Academy of Pediatrics, 1997).
- High compliance of the airway makes it very susceptible to dynamic collapse when it is obstructed (Wittenborg *et al.*, 1967).
- There is high oxygen demand because of high metabolic rate – per kg weight, oxygen consumption in infants is twice that in adults (Cross *et al.*, 1957).
- The ribs and intercostal cartilage are very compliant and can fail to support breathing (Mansell *et al.*, 1972).
- Tidal volume is almost totally dependent upon movement of the diaphragm and any condition that impedes this, e.g. gastric distension, can compromise breathing (American Academy of Pediatrics, 1997).

Causes of airway obstruction

Causes of airway obstruction include (European Resuscitation Council, 1998):

- displaced tongue – causes include unconsciousness, cardiac arrest and trauma
- fluid – e.g. vomit, secretions and blood
- foreign body
- laryngeal oedema – causes include anaphylaxis and infection
- bronchospasm – causes include asthma, foreign body and anaphylaxis
- trauma
- pulmonary oedema – causes include cardiac failure, anaphylaxis and near drowning.

Recognition of airway obstruction

Whatever the cause of airway obstruction, prompt recognition and effective management are essential. Recognition is best achieved by following the familiar look, listen and feel approach (Resuscitation Council (UK), 2000c):

Look   for movements of the chest and abdomen.

Listen   at the mouth and nose for airflow.

Feel   at the mouth and nose for airflow.

Airway obstruction can be partial or complete, and can occur at any level from the nose and mouth down to the trachea (European Resuscitation Council, 1998).

Partial airway obstruction

Partial airway obstruction is usually characterized by noisy breathing:

- **gurgling** – presence of fluid, e.g. secretions, in the main airways
- **snoring** – partial occlusion of the pharynx by the tongue
- **crowing** – laryngeal spasm
- **inspiratory stridor** – upper airway obstruction (at or above the level of the larynx), e.g. foreign body, croup
- **expiratory wheeze** – lower airway obstruction, e.g. asthma.

Complete airway obstruction

Complete airway obstruction in a child who is making respiratory efforts is characterized by paradoxical chest and abdominal movements ('see-saw' breathing) – on trying to breathe in, the chest is drawn inwards and the abdomen expands, the opposite happening when trying to breathe out.

Simple techniques to open and clear the airway

The airway in an unconscious child can easily become obstructed by a combination of flexion of the neck, relaxation of the jaw, displacement of the tongue against the posterior wall of the pharynx and collapse of the hypopharynx (Hudgel and Hendricks, 1988; Abernethy *et al.*, 1990). In some cases, just opening the airway may revive the child.

Head tilt/chin lift

The airway can be opened by tilting the head and lifting the chin. This will help to open the airway and bring the tongue forward from the posterior wall of the pharynx (the tongue is the most common cause of airway obstruction in an unconscious child; Ruben *et al.*, 1961). The neutral position in an infant (Fig. 5.1a) and the 'sniffing the morning air' position in a child (Fig. 5.1b) are recommended (ALSG, 2001). Care should be taken not to press on the soft tissues under the chin as this may obstruct the airway. Blind finger sweeps are not recommended.

Jaw thrust

Although cervical spine injuries are rare in infants and children (American Academy of Pediatrics, 1997), if there is a history of trauma, the jaw thrust

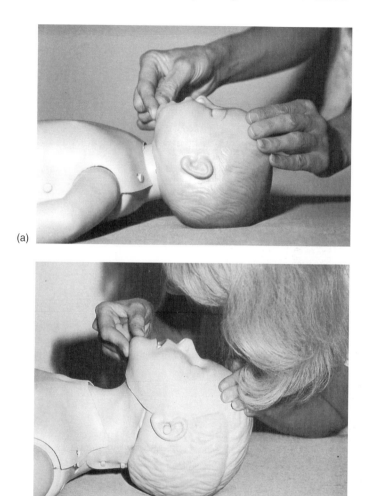

(a)

(b)

Fig. 5.1   Head tilt/chin lift: (a) neutral position in a baby; (b) sniffing the morning air position in a child.

rather than head tilt/chin lift is recommended (ALSG, 2001). Position two to three fingers under each side of the lower jaw at its angle and lift upwards and outwards (American Academy of Pediatrics, 1997). This should be accompanied by manual in-line immobilization of the head and neck by an assistant (Nolan and Parr, 1997).

Suction

When obstruction is caused by vomit, secretions, etc., simple BLS man-oeuvres such as placing the child in the lateral position and finger sweeps under direct vision can help to clear the airway.

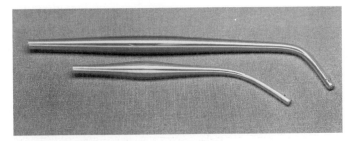

Fig. 5.2 Rigid wide-bore (Yankauer) suction catheter.

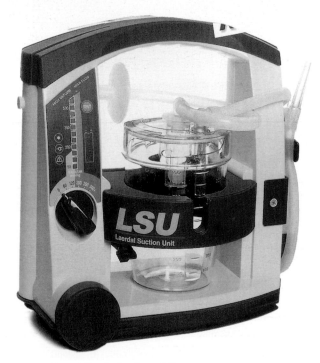

Fig. 5.3 Portable suction device (Laerdal).

A wide-bore rigid (Yankauer) catheter (Fig. 5.2) can provide rapid suction of large volumes of fluid from the mouth and pharynx. A flexible catheter is particularly useful for suctioning down an oropharyngeal airway, nasopharyngeal airway and tracheal tube. In order to minimize deoxygenation, suction should last no longer than 10 seconds (Idris *et al.*, 1996).

A wall suction device is ideal for suction at the bedside. There are also a number of portable suction devices currently available which are ideal in some situations, e.g. during patient transfer. Laerdal's Premier Suction Unit (Fig. 5.3) is light and durable. It has a variable vacuum regulator

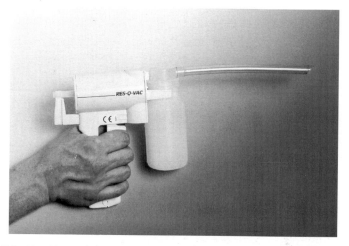

Fig. 5.4   Hand-held suction device (Timesco of London).

which makes it ideal for both paediatric and adult use. It can be operated by either a battery or an external power source. It also has a specially designed filter to protect the collection vessel. A hand-held suction device (Fig. 5.4) is particularly useful in the primary care setting.

Principles of cricoid pressure

Cricoid pressure was first described by Sellick, who advocated its use during the induction of anaesthesia to reduce the incidence of aspiration of gastric contents (Sellick, 1961).

The high incidence of gastric inflation (Berg *et al.*, 1998) and pulmonary aspiration during cardiac arrests (Lawes and Baskett, 1987) emphasizes the need for all practitioners to be aware of the value of cricoid pressure during CPR and be competent and safe at providing it. It is also sometimes useful during tracheal intubation as it can facilitate visualization of the vocal cords.

Mode of action

By occluding the lumen of the oesophagus, cricoid pressure will help to prevent regurgitation and aspiration of gastric contents and gastric inflation during ventilation, particularly when a bag/valve/mask device is used (Petito and Russell, 1988; Moynihan *et al.*, 1993).

Technique

1. Palpate a prominent horizontal band below the thyroid cartilage (Adam's apple) and cricothyroid membrane.

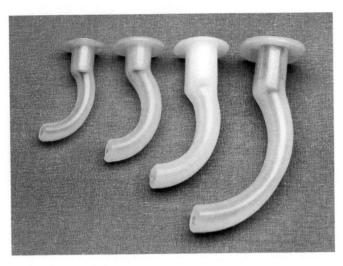

Fig. 5.5   Oropharyngeal airways.

2. Apply backward pressure on the cricoid using one fingertip in infants and the thumb and index finger in children. This will help to obstruct the lumen of the oesophagus lying posteriorly (if there is a suspected cervical spine injury, counter-pressure may be applied to the back of the neck to reduce the movement of the cervical spine (Resuscitation Council (UK), 2000a)).
3. Release cricoid pressure only when a tracheal tube protects the airway (or if the child actively vomits).

Cautions

Cricoid pressure should not be applied during active vomiting because there is a risk of damage to the oesophagus (Resuscitation Council (UK), 2000a). Too much pressure may compress and obstruct the trachea and could distort upper airway anatomy (Hartsilver and Vanner, 2000), making tracheal intubation difficult.

Oropharyngeal and nasopharyngeal airways

Oropharyngeal (Guedel) and nasopharyngeal airways are useful adjuncts because they can provide an artificial passage for airflow by separating the posterior pharyngeal wall from the tongue. Each type is discussed below.

Oropharyngeal airway

The oropharyngeal airway (Fig. 5.5) can be used when there is obstruction of the upper airway because of displacement of the tongue backwards and

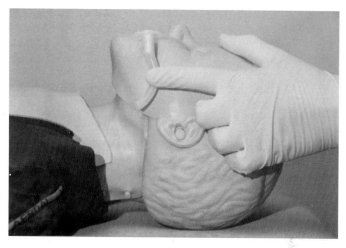

Fig. 5.6 Oropharyngeal airway insertion: estimating the correct size of airway.

when glossopharyngeal and laryngeal reflexes are absent. However, it is usually only used when head tilt and chin lift have failed to provide a clear airway (American Academy of Pediatrics, 1997). It should not be used if the child is not completely unconscious as it may induce vomiting and laryngospasm (Mehta, 1990).

It is important to ensure the correct size is used because:

- if it is too big it may actually block the airway, hinder the use of a face-mask and damage laryngeal structures
- if it is too small it may block the airway by pushing the tongue back.

An appropriately sized airway is one that holds the tongue in the normal anatomical position and follows its natural curvature (Idris *et al.*, 1996). The curved body of the oropharyngeal airway is designed to fit over the back of the tongue. The correct size can be estimated by placing the airway against the face and measuring it from the corner of the mouth to the angle of the jaw (Fig. 5.6) (American Academy of Pediatrics, 1997). Various sizes of oropharyngeal airways are currently available (Fig. 5.5).

It is also important to insert the airway correctly in order to avoid unnecessary trauma to the delicate tissues in the mouth and inadvertently blocking the airway.

In older children, the oropharyngeal airway (lubricated if possible) can be inserted into the mouth in the inverted position (the curved part of the airway will help depress the tongue and prevent it from being pushed posteriorly) and, as it passes over the soft palate, rotated through 180 degrees (ALSG, 2001). Following insertion of the airway, patency of the airway should be checked and head tilt/chin lift maintained.

In infants, the oropharyngeal airway (lubricated if possible) should be inserted 'right side up' with the tongue depressed out of the way

(ALSG, 2001) – if inserted in the inverted position it may damage the soft palate. Following insertion, the patency of the airway should be checked and head tilt/chin lift maintained.

Nasopharyngeal airway

The nasopharyngeal airway is preferable if the child is semi-conscious because the risk of gagging, vomiting and laryngospasm is minimal. It is less likely to induce gagging than an oropharyngeal airway and it can be used in a semi-conscious or conscious child when the airway is at risk of being compromised.

It is contraindicated if there is a suspected base of skull fracture, as it may penetrate the cranial fossa (Muzzi *et al.*, 1991).

Insertion may damage the mucosal lining of the nasal airway, resulting in bleeding. The correct size should be used and, prior to insertion, a safety pin should be securely inserted into the flange to prevent inhalation of the airway.

It is important to estimate the correct length. If it is too short it will be ineffective, and if it is too long it may enter the oesophagus causing distension and hypoventilation, or may stimulate the laryngeal or glosso-pharyngeal reflexes causing laryngospasm and vomiting.

The correct length of the nasopharyngeal airway is one that equates with the distance from the tip of the nose to the tragus of the ear (American Academy of Pediatrics, 1997). The correct width is one that does not cause sustained blanching of the alae nasi (American Academy of Pediatrics, 1997).

Paediatric-sized nasopharyngeal airways are commercially available, or a shortened tracheal tube may be used (ALSG, 2001). Following lubrication, the airway should be gently inserted through the nostril in a posterior direction perpendicular to the plane of the child's face (American Academy of Pediatrics, 1997). It is important to put the 15 mm adapter back into the tracheal tube to avoid accidental advancement of the tube past the nares.

Reassess the airway and check for patency and adequacy of ventilation. Continue to maintain correct alignment of the airway and chin lift as necessary and monitor the patency of the airway. Suction as necessary.

Principles of tracheal intubation

Tracheal intubation is the best method of securing the upper airway (Zideman and Spearpoint, 1999). It enables suction of the trachea and lower airways, delivery of high concentrations of inspired oxygen and facilitates mechanical ventilation.

The risk of gastric distension, regurgitation and aspiration of gastric contents, which are not uncommon during BLS, is minimized. However, as the technique can be difficult and sometimes hazardous, regular experience in its use is required.

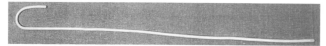

Fig. 5.7   Stylet.

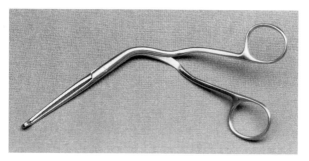

Fig. 5.8   Magill's forceps.

Indications

Indications for tracheal intubation include:

- ineffective ventilation
- high peak inspiratory pressures required
- prolonged ventilation
- transfer.

Equipment

A suggested list of equipment includes:

- laryngoscope ×2, in working order with appropriate blades
- tracheal tube of estimated size, together with one 0.5 mm smaller and one 0.5 mm larger; uncuffed tubes tend to be used in children <8 years of age so as not to cause oedema at the cricoid ring (ALSG, 2001)
- suction source, including a Yankauer (rigid) suction catheter and a suction catheter of appropriate size to suction down the tracheal tube
- oxygen source
- tape to secure the tube
- stylet (Fig. 5.7)
- ventilation device, e.g. bag/valve/mask
- stethoscope
- Magill's forceps (Fig. 5.8).

Tracheal tubes

Tracheal tubes (Fig. 5.9) come in a variety of different designs and sizes. A standard 15 mm adapter is connected to the proximal end, enabling the attachment of a ventilatory device.

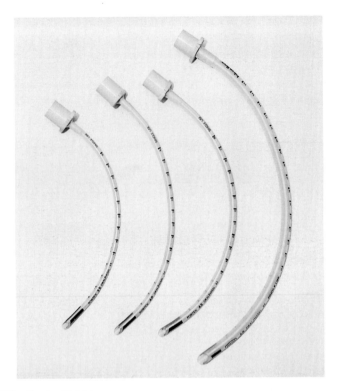

Fig. 5.9 Tracheal tubes.

Uncuffed tracheal tubes are commonly used in preference to cuffed tubes in children <8 years so as not to cause oedema at the cricoid ring (ALSG, 2001). Cuffed tubes are occasionally used in children <8 years of age, particularly if higher inspiratory pressures are required, e.g. in asthma (American Heart Association, 2000). However, as long as cuff pressure is closely monitored, complication rates of cuffed and uncuffed tubes are similar (Deakers *et al.*, 1994; Khine *et al.*, 1997).

The tracheal tube should have distance markers (cms) which provide a point of reference during intubation and, following intubation, facilitate the early detection of tube migration.

The correct size of tracheal tube (internal diameter in mm) can be estimated by:

- Referring to a paediatric resuscitation chart or a length-based resuscitation tape – body length is better than body weight at predicting correct tube size (Luten *et al.*, 1992).
- Using a recognized formula. A suggested formula for children over 1 year old is (age/4) +4 (ALSG, 2001), e.g. the estimated internal diameter for an 8-year-old is (8/4) +4 = 6 mm. There is no formula as such for

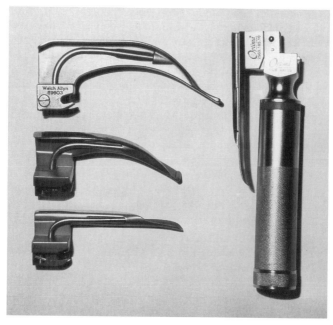

Fig. 5.10 Laryngoscope and selection of blades.

infants <1 year, but diameters of 3.0/3.5 mm at birth and 3.5/4.0 mm at 6 months usually suffice.

- Measuring the size of the little finger – caution is needed as this method can be unreliable (Luten *et al.*, 1992).

A suggested formula for estimating the correct length (cm) of an oral tracheal tube is (age/2) + 12 (ALSG, 2001).

Laryngoscope

The laryngoscope consists of a handle containing batteries and a blade with a light source. In modern fibreoptic laryngoscopes, the bulb is situated in the top of the handle rather than in the blade itself – this design feature is preferable because the bulb is secure and protected and the blade can easily be cleaned after use.

There are two main designs of laryngoscope blade (Fig. 5.10) for use in children:

Straight blade   This is preferred for infants and small children because it provides better visualization of the relatively cephalad and anterior glottis (American Academy of Pediatrics, 1997). It is designed to pass over the epiglottis and rest at the opening of the glottis. Blade traction (upwards and forwards along the line of the handle) will lift the base of the tongue and the epiglottis anteriorly and expose the glottis (American Heart Association, 2000).

Curved blade This is preferred for older children because the wider base and flange facilitates tongue displacement and improves visualization of the glottis (American Academy of Pediatrics, 1997). The tip of the blade should rest in the vallecula (space between the base of the tongue and the epiglottis). Blade traction (upwards and forwards along the line of the handle) will then displace the base of the tongue anteriorly and expose the glottis (American Heart Association, 2000).

The advantage of advancing the blade past the epiglottis is that the latter will then not obscure the visualization of the vocal cords; the advantage of stopping short of the epiglottis is that it will cause less stimulation and is therefore less likely to cause laryngospasm (ALSG, 2001). Inserting the blade first into the oesophagus and then slowly withdrawing it until the glottis is visualized can cause laryngeal trauma and is not recommended (American Academy of Pediatrics, 1997).

It is possible to successfully intubate with a blade that is too long, but not with one that is too short (ALSG, 2001).

Procedure for tracheal intubation

1. Ensure that access to the child's head is not restricted. Move the bed away from the wall and remove the backrest if applicable.
2. Assemble the necessary equipment and check to see if it is in good working order.
3. Position yourself at the child's head end with the feet in the walk/stand position (Resuscitation Council (UK), 2001).
4. Correctly position the head (the axes of the mouth, pharynx and trachea should be aligned in order to be able to directly visualize the glottis). In a child of >2 years, place the head on a small pillow. This will slightly flex the neck and bring the larynx into optimum alignment for tracheal intubation. In infants and children <2 years, the head should be placed on a flat surface – a pillow is not required, though a small rolled-up towel under the shoulders is sometimes used to maintain the position. If the neck is over-extended this will lift the glottis out of the line of sight and the trachea may become obstructed. Difficulties in visualization will also occur if the neck is flexed.
5. If possible, pre-oxygenate the child for a minimum of 15 seconds.
6. Hold the laryngoscope in the left hand (irrespective of handedness). While the right hand opens the child's mouth, gently insert the laryngoscope into the right-hand corner ensuring that the lower lip is not caught between the teeth and the blade.
7. Slide the laryngoscope blade into the mouth, sweeping the tongue to the left in the process.
8. Advance the tip of the blade. If a curved blade is used, it is usually positioned in the vallecula, the area between the back of the tongue and the

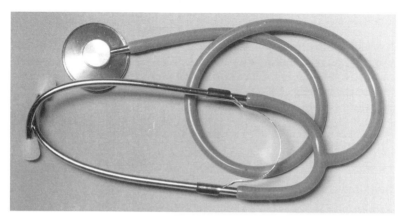

Fig. 5.11   Auscultate the chest for air entry.

base of the epiglottis. If a straight blade is used, it is usually positioned just past the epiglottis.

9. Lift the laryngoscope upwards in the line of the handle. This should lift the epiglottis out of the way and expose the glottis and vocal cords. Suction if necessary.
10. Insert the tracheal tube from the right-hand side of the mouth through the vocal cords, positioning the black marker on the tracheal tube just below the glottic opening.
11. Connect to a self-inflating bag and ventilate. In older children, a catheter mount is sometimes also attached to allow greater movement of the bag. However, it should be used with caution because it does increase the dead space.
12. Confirm correct tube placement (see below).
13. Secure the tube, continue ventilation and continually reassess tube position. Excessive head movement can displace the tube: the tube can be displaced further into and out of the airway by head flexion and head extension respectively (Hartrey and Kestin, 1995).
14. Adopt a comfortable position and avoid prolonged static postures (Resuscitation Council (UK), 2001).

Confirming correct tube placement

It is important to confirm correct tube placement:

- Look for bilateral and symmetrical chest movement.
- Auscultate (Fig. 5.11) the chest over the axillae for breath sounds and listen over the stomach – breath sounds should be absent over the upper abdomen (Andersen and Schultz-Lebahn, 1994).
- Check end-tidal CO_2 – after six ventilations, a positive colour change or the presence of an exhaled CO_2 waveform confirms the position of the

tube (Bhende *et al.*, 1992). However, this method may not be helpful during a cardiac arrest because the absence of a positive colour change or an exhaled CO_2 waveform does not necessarily equate with oesophageal intubation – limited pulmonary blood flow can result in undetectable exhaled CO_2 despite correct tracheal tube placement (Bhende and Thompson, 1995).

• Perform a chest X-ray.

If in doubt, take it out.

Ineffective ventilation following tracheal intubation

Ventilation may not be established effectively after intubation or it may become ineffective after a variable period. The main causes of this can be described by the acronym DOPE:

• Displaced tube – into either pharynx/oesophagus, or right/left main bronchus
• Obstructed tube – vomit, blood, secretions or kinked tube
• Pneumothorax
• Equipment failure.

These problems should be recognized and diagnosed by the checks that routinely follow intubation.

Principles of oxygen delivery and ventilation

NB: The most common cause of failure to ventilate is improper positioning of the head and chin (Idris *et al.*, 1996).

Mouth-to-mouth ventilation has been discussed in Chapter 4. Mouth-to-mask ventilation and ventilation with a bag/valve/mask device is described below.

Mouth-to-mask ventilation (pocket mask)

A well-fitting pocket mask (Fig. 5.12) used by trained rescuers is an effective method of ventilation (Safar, 1974). It can be used in adults and children and, when used upside-down, in infants (ALSG, 2001). Most are transparent, thus enabling prompt detection of any vomit or blood in the airway. Some have a nipple for the attachment of supplementary oxygen. A one-way valve directs the child's expired air away from the rescuer.

Method

1. Move the bed away from the wall and remove the backrest if applicable (if a cot or resuscitaire, ensure easy access). Ensure the brakes are on.

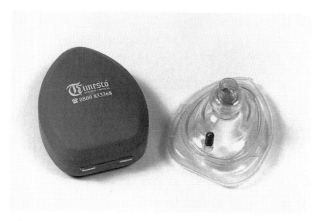

Fig. 5.12   Pocket mask (Timesco of London).

2. Position yourself at the top of the bed facing the child, with the feet in a walk/stand position.
3. If available, attach oxygen to the nipple at a flow rate of 10 litres per minute. This will allow the delivery of up to 50% oxygen (Lawrence and Sivaneswaran, 1985).
4. Ensure that the child is supine and tilt the head back. A pillow under the head and shoulders can help to maintain this position.
5. Apply the mask to the face, pressing down with the thumbs.
6. Lift the chin into the mask by applying pressure behind the angles of the jaw.
7. Ventilate the patient with sufficient air to cause visible chest rise. Observe for chest rise and fall.
8. Adopt a comfortable position for ventilation and avoid static postures.

Principles of bag/valve/mask ventilation

The facemask

Facemasks come in a variety of different shapes, sizes and materials. For infants the popular circular masks (Fig. 5.13) are generally preferred. Advantages of these masks include:

- soft cushioned rim that will conform to the contour of the baby's face making it easier to form the seal that is essential for effective lung inflation
- made of transparent silicone so that secretions etc. can be easily seen
- minimal dead space.

Rigid triangular masks are not recommended as they are more prone to air leakage (Palme *et al.*, 1985). In older children, the traditional triangular shaped mask (Fig. 5.14) is recommended. It is important to ensure that the soft cushioned rim is adequately inflated.

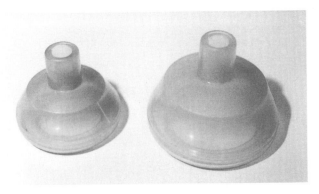

Fig. 5.13   Round resuscitation facemasks.

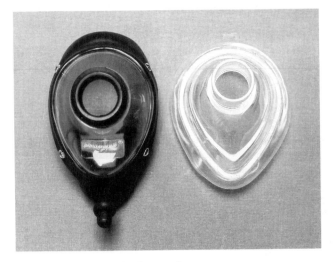

Fig. 5.14   Triangular resuscitation facemasks.

When choosing a mask, make sure that it is of an appropriate size and that it will fit snugly over both mouth and nose but neither cause pressure on the eyes nor create an air leak by overriding the chin.

The self-inflating bag

There are a number of different makes of self-inflating bag available, but they all work on the same principle. Personnel using this device ought to be familiar with its structure and function. The self-inflating bag (Fig. 5.15) consists of the following components:

The bag (A)   Different bag sizes are available. The 500-ml bag (Fig. 5.16) should be used for the resuscitation of infants and small children. It will reinflate by recoil after being squeezed, even if no gas is entering. The

Pressure relief
valve (G)

Outlet
valve (F)

The bag (A)   Air inlet (B)

Oxygen reservoir
valve (I)

Oxygen reservoir

Patient outlet (E)

Inlet valve (H)

Oxygen inlet (C)

Oxygen reservoir
bag (D)

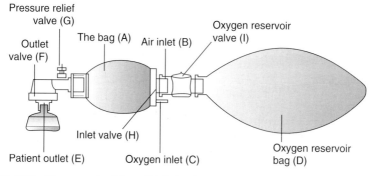

Fig. 5.15   Components of the self-inflating bag.

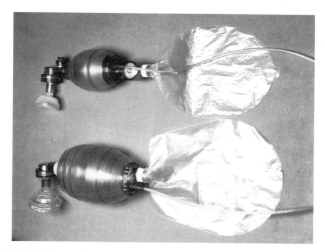

Fig. 5.16   Self-inflating bags: 500 ml (above) and 150 ml (below).

1500-ml (adult) bag (Fig. 5.16) is generally only used in older children. However, it could be used (with extreme care) in infants (Tendrup *et al.*, 1989). The 250-ml (neonatal) bag is considered too small for infant resuscitation (Field *et al.*, 1986).

The air inlet (B)   Oxygen is sucked through the air inlet if the oxygen reservoir bag is full and attached. If it is not attached, air will be sucked through.

The oxygen inlet (C)   Oxygen is delivered to the bag here at a recommended rate of 10 litres per minute (if the oxygen tubing is connected and the flowmeter turned on).

The reservoir bag (D)   With an oxygen flow rate of 10 litres per minute, this will increase the oxygen concentration delivered to the baby to approximately 85% (Resuscitation Council (UK), 2000a). Oxygen is allowed to fill the reservoir during expiration, enabling the rapid refilling of the bag.

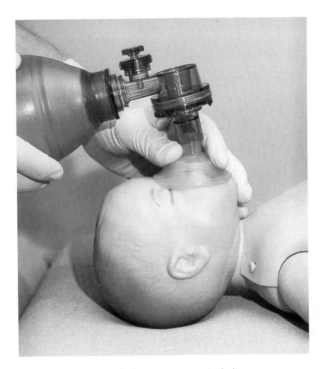

Fig. 5.17   Bag/valve/mask ventilation: one-person technique.

The patient outlet (E)   This connects directly to the facemask or the tracheal tube adapter.

The outlet valve (F)   This is situated between the bag and patient outlet; it opens when the bag is squeezed allowing gas through to the child.

The pressure relief valve (G)   This is situated between the bag and outlet valve; it opens at about 30–40 cmH$_2$O preventing very high pressures being generated which could cause a pneumothorax. However, there must be an override feature so that high pressures can be generated if required in order to achieve chest rise (Hirschman and Kravath, 1982). Higher pressures may be required if there is upper or lower airway obstruction or if there is poor lung compliance – in these situations a pressure relief valve may prevent the delivery of a sufficient tidal volume (Finer *et al.*, 1986).

The inlet valve (H)   This is situated between the bag and the air inlet; it allows air to enter the bag during refilling but prevents exit during squeezing.

The oxygen reservoir valve (I)   This allows excess oxygen to escape.

Although the bag/valve/mask device does allow the delivery of higher concentrations of oxygen, its use by one person (Fig. 5.17) requires considerable

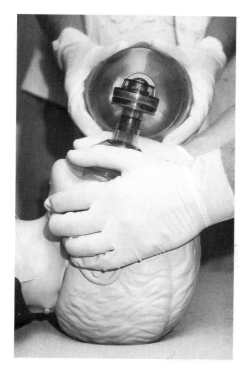

Fig. 5.18 Bag/valve/mask ventilation: two-person technique.

skill and may in fact be ineffective (Harrison and Maull, 1982; Hess and Baran, 1985).

Consequently, a two-person technique is recommended (Hess and Baran, 1985; Jesudian *et al.*, 1985), one person to open the airway and ensure a good seal with the mask while the other squeezes the bag (Fig. 5.18). An oxygen reservoir bag should ideally be used as this will enable the delivery of high concentrations of oxygen.

Method
1. Move the bed away from the wall and remove the backrest if applicable. Ensure the brakes on the bed are on.
2. Position yourself at the top of the bed facing the child, with the feet in a walk/stand position.
3. Select an appropriate size of mask. This should comfortably cover the mouth and nose. It should not cover the eyes or override the chin. The mask should be transparent, thus enabling prompt detection of any vomit or blood in the airway. It should also have a soft pliable edge to facilitate achieving a good seal with the face.
4. Select an appropriately sized bag.

5. Ensure that the oxygen reservoir bag is attached and connect oxygen at a flow rate of 10–15 litres per minute (Finer *et al.*, 1986). This will usually achieve an inspired oxygen concentration of approximately 85% (Resuscitation Council (UK), 2000a).
6. Ensure that the child is supine. The first rescuer should tilt the head back, and apply the mask to the face, pressing down on it with the thumbs. The chin should then be lifted into the mask by applying pressure behind the angles of the jaw. An open airway and an adequate facemask seal should now be achieved. In a child, a pillow under the head and shoulders can help to maintain this position. In an infant and smaller child, a rolled-up blanket under the shoulders may help.
7. Ask your colleague, who should be positioned to the side of the bed, to slowly squeeze the bag/valve device (not the oxygen reservoir bag) with sufficient air to cause visible chest rise.
8. Observe for chest rise and fall. If the chest does not rise recheck the patency of the airway. Slight readjustment may be all that is required.
9. Adopt a comfortable position for ventilation and avoid static postures. Supporting your weight by resting your elbows on the bed may help.

If ventilation is judged ineffective, recheck airway patency and the facemask seal. Consider equipment failure. In each case take appropriate action. If the lungs are known to be stiff, a higher inflation pressure can be tried by disabling the pressure relief valve.

Gastric inflation
Unless the child's airway is secured with a tracheal tube, ventilation carries a high risk of gastric inflation, regurgitation of gastric contents and pulmonary aspiration (Melker, 1985). Gastric inflation can also limit effective ventilation (Berg *et al.*, 1998). There is an increased risk of gastric inflation when:

- inflation pressures and volumes are high
- the head and neck are not aligned
- the airway is not patent
- the oesophageal sphincter is incompetent.

To minimize the risk of gastric inflation the following is recommended:

- deliver inflations slowly over 1–2 seconds
- deliver a tidal volume to achieve chest rise
- ensure a patent airway
- apply cricoid pressure – reduces gastric inflation (Moynihan *et al.*, 1993) and may prevent regurgitation and aspiration of gastric contents.

(If gastric distension develops, the stomach should be decompressed with a nasogastric tube (American Heart Association, 2000).)

Summary

Effective airway management and ventilation are essential aspects of paediatric resuscitation. Relevant anatomy and physiology, causes and recognition of airway obstruction have been discussed. Simple techniques to open and clear the airway, together with the principles of cricoid pressure have been described. The role of oropharyngeal/nasopharyngeal/laryngeal mask airways has been discussed. The procedure for tracheal intubation and the principles of ventilation have been highlighted.

Chapter 6

Cardiac monitoring and ECG recognition

Introduction

Although primary cardiac events are uncommon in children, cardiac monitoring is nevertheless still an important aspect of paediatric advanced life support. Once the presenting ECG rhythm has been identified, the appropriate treatment can then be administered. Poor technique, however, can lead to an inaccurate ECG trace and mistaken diagnosis. A sound knowledge of the principles of cardiac monitoring is therefore paramount.

An understanding of the principles of ECG recognition is also important. It will enable the identification of abnormal ECG rhythms which may compromise cardiac output, precede or be associated with cardiac arrest, or complicate recovery after successful CPR. An understanding of the basic principles of ECG recognition is therefore also essential.

The aim of this chapter is to understand the principles of cardiac monitoring and ECG recognition.

Objectives

At the end of this chapter the reader will be able to:

- describe the conduction system of the heart
- describe the ECG and its relation to cardiac contraction
- describe a suggested ECG electrode placement for cardiac monitoring
- state the problems that can be encountered with cardiac monitoring
- outline a simple three-stage approach to ECG recognition
- recognize sinus bradycardia, sinus tachycardia, supraventricular tachycardia and ventricular tachycardia.

The conduction system of the heart

The heart possesses specialized muscle cells that initiate and conduct electrical impulses resulting in myocardial contraction. This conduction system (Fig. 6.1) comprises the following:

- sinus node (sinoatrial or SA node)
- atrioventricular node or junction

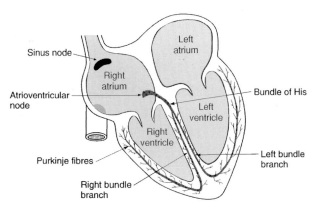

Fig. 6.1 Conduction system of the heart.

- bundle of His
- bundle branches (right and left)
- Purkinje fibres.

Nervous control of the heart rate

The sinus node normally acts as the pacemaker for myocardial contraction.
The rate at which it fires is dependent upon the autonomic nervous system:

- *parasympathetic or vagus nerve* – an increase in activity slows down the heart rate while a decrease in activity speeds up the heart rate; atropine blocks the vagus nerve causing an increase in heart rate
- *sympathetic nerve* – prepares the body for 'fight and flight' and will result in an increase in heart rate and an increase in the force of myocardial contraction.

The ECG and its relation to cardiac contraction

(Fig. 6.2)

1. The sinus node fires and the electrical impulse spreads across the atria causing atrial contraction (P wave).
2. On arriving at the atrioventricular node, the impulse is delayed to allow the atria time to fully contract and eject blood into the ventricles. This brief period of absent electrical activity is represented on the ECG by a straight (isoelectric) line between the end of the P wave and the beginning of the QRS complex.
3. The impulse is then conducted to the ventricles through the bundle of His, right and left bundle branches and Purkinje fibres causing ventricular depolarization and contraction (QRS complex).
4. The ventricles then repolarize (T wave).

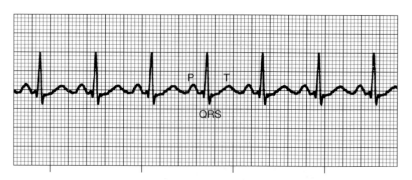

Fig. 6.2   ECG and its relation to cardiac contraction.

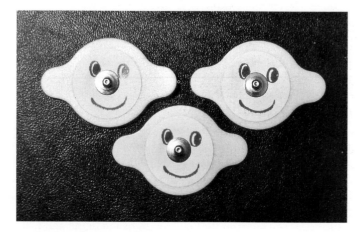

Fig. 6.3   Paediatric ECG electrodes.

Suggested ECG electrode placement for cardiac monitoring

During paediatric resuscitation, lead II is the best lead for cardiac monitoring. The monitor/defibrillator should be switched on, lead II should be selected and the ECG electrodes (Fig. 6.3) should be positioned as follows:

- *red* on the right shoulder
- *yellow* on the left shoulder
- *green* on the left upper abdominal wall.

This ECG electrode placement (Fig. 6.4) benefits from reduced muscle interference and will not hinder paddle placement if defibrillation is required.

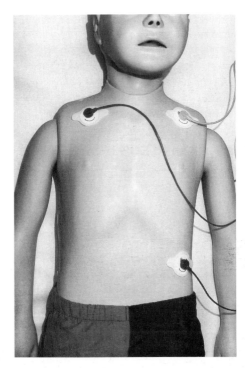

Fig. 6.4   Suggested placement of ECG electrodes during resuscitation.

Sometimes in the emergency setting, initial ECG monitoring is established using the defibrillator paddles. Select 'Paddles' setting on the defibrillator and apply gel pads and paddles to chest (see Fig. 7.6, p. 83).

Problems encountered with cardiac monitoring

'Straight line' ECG trace   Check the child, the monitoring lead selected (normally lead II), ECG gain, ECG leads and electrodes. NB: Asystole is rarely a straight line.

Poor-quality ECG trace   Check all the connections and the brightness display. Ensure that the electrodes are correctly attached, are 'in-date' and that the gel sponge is moist, not dry (Perez, 1996). Ensure that the skin where the electrodes are attached is dry.

Interference and artefacts   Poor electrode contact, child movement, CPR and electrical interference, e.g. from bedside infusion pumps, can cause the ECG trace to be 'fuzzy'. Apply the electrodes over bone rather than muscle to minimize interference (Resuscitation Council (UK), 2000b).

Wandering baseline   An ECG trace going up and down is usually caused by child movement or simply by ventilation. Reposition the electrodes away from the lower ribs (Meltzer, 1983).

Small ECG complexes   The most likely cause of small and unrecognizable ECG complexes is a technical problem; check that the ECG gain is adequate and that the appropriate ECG monitoring lead (lead II) is selected on the monitor.

Incorrect heart rate display   Causes include small QRS complexes, large T waves, muscle movement and interference. Ensure that the ECG trace is reliable.

Three-stage approach to ECG recognition

The Advanced Life Support Group (ALSG) (2001) recommend the following three-stage approach to ECG recognition:

- estimation of the QRS rate
- assessment of the QRS rhythm
- measurement of the QRS width.

Estimation of the QRS rate

Estimate the QRS rate by counting the number of large (1 cm) squares between adjacent QRS complexes and dividing it into 300, e.g. the QRS rate in Figure 6.2 is about 150 (300/2). Care should be taken if the QRS rate is irregular. Establish whether the QRS rate is normal, abnormally fast or abnormally slow. The normal ranges for heart rate are dependent upon the child's age (see Table 3.2).

Assessment of the QRS rhythm

Establish whether the QRS rhythm is regular or irregular by carefully comparing the R–R intervals at different sections on the ECG rhythm strip.

Measurement of the QRS width

Measure the QRS width. The normal width is 2.5 small squares (0.10 seconds) or less. If the width is broad (>2.5 small squares), the rhythm may be ventricular in origin or supraventricular in origin, but transmitted with aberrant conduction. A broad complex tachycardia is more likely to be ventricular in origin.

Sinus rhythm is the normal rhythm (Fig. 6.2), indicating that the impulse is initiated by the SA node at a normal rate for the child's age and is conducted down the normal conduction pathways without being delayed.

Recognition of sinus bradycardia, sinus tachycardia, supraventricular tachycardia and ventricular tachycardia

Sinus bradycardia

Sinus bradycardia (Fig. 6.5) can be defined as a rate of sinus node discharge slower than the normal for the child's age (see Table 3.2). It is usually

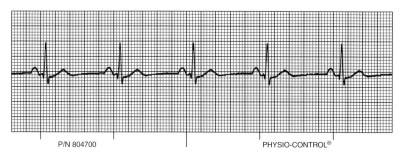

P/N 804700　　　　　　　　　　　　　PHYSIO-CONTROL®

Fig. 6.5　Sinus bradycardia.

a pre-terminal sign in children with respiratory or circulatory failure. The most common cause is hypoxaemia. Other causes include acidosis, hypothermia, raised intracranial pressure and vagal stimulation, e.g. during suction or tracheal intubation. In small infants (< 6 months), as cardiac output is more dependent upon the heart rate, a bradycardia is more likely to cause symptoms (American Heart Association, 2000).

Sinus tachycardia

Sinus tachycardia (Fig. 6.6) can be defined as a rate of sinus node discharge faster than the normal for the child's age (see Table 3.2). Causes include anxiety, pyrexia, pain, blood loss, sepsis and shock (American Academy of Pediatrics, 2000). Treatment is aimed at identifying and, if possible, treating the cause.

Supraventricular tachycardia

Supraventricular tachycardia (SVT) (Fig. 6.7) is the most common non-arrest cardiac arrhythmia in children and the most common cardiac arrhythmia in infants that produces cardiovascular instability (ALSG, 2001). The ventricular rate in SVT is typically > 220 and the QRS complexes are narrow. Ideally a 12-lead ECG should be recorded to help confirm diagnosis.

Differentiating between sinus tachycardia and SVT can sometimes be difficult. The ALSG (2001) suggest that the following characteristics will assist correct ECG interpretation:

- Ventricular rate: sinus tachycardia < 200; SVT > 220
- If P waves can be identified: upright in leads I and AVF (sinus tachycardia); negative in II, III and AVF (SVT)
- Rate and regularity: varies in sinus tachycardia; constant in SVT
- Onset and termination: gradual in sinus tachycardia; abrupt in SVT
- History of shock is usually present with sinus tachycardia.

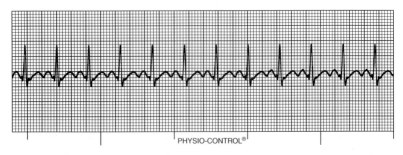

Fig. 6.6   Sinus tachycardia.

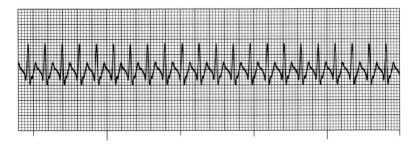

Fig. 6.7   Supraventricular tachycardia.

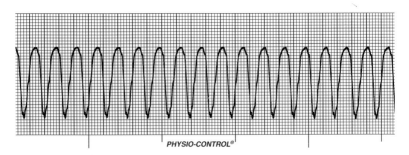

Fig. 6.8   Ventricular tachycardia.

The child's age, ventricular rate, duration of SVT and ventricular function prior to the onset all influence the haemodynamic effect of SVT (American Heart Association, 2000).

Ventricular tachycardia

Ventricular tachycardia (Fig. 6.8), a rare cardiac arrhythmia in childhood, is characterized by a rapid QRS rate and wide QRS complexes. Causes include poisoning, hyperkalaemia and cardiac surgery. Sometimes it will result in a loss of cardiac output, requiring urgent defibrillation.

If possible, a 12-lead ECG should be recorded and analysed with the help of a paediatric cardiologist (by fax if necessary) (ALSG, 2001).

Summary

Cardiac monitoring and ECG recognition form an integral part of paediatric advanced life support. The principles of accurate cardiac monitoring have been discussed. A system to interpret ECGs has been described.

Chapter 7

Defibrillation

Introduction

Defibrillation is the delivery of an electrical current to the myocardium to terminate ventricular fibrillation. Although first described in 1899, it was not until 1956 that the first external defibrillation in a human was reported (Zoll *et al.*, 1956).

Although defibrillation is rare in the paediatric arrest situation, when it is indicated it is important to ensure that it is performed rapidly, safely and effectively. Knowledge of the principles of defibrillation is therefore required.

The aim of this chapter is to understand the principles of defibrillation.

Objectives

At the end of this chapter the reader will be able to:

- describe ventricular fibrillation
- discuss the physiology of defibrillation
- outline the factors affecting successful defibrillation
- discuss the safety issues related to defibrillation
- describe the procedure for manual defibrillation
- describe the procedure for automated external defibrillation
- describe the procedure for emergency synchronized cardioversion
- discuss the new technological advances in defibrillation.

Ventricular fibrillation

'The cardiac pump is thrown out of gear, and the last of its vital energy is dissipated in a violent and prolonged turmoil of fruitless activity in the ventricular walls' (McWilliam, 1889).

In ventricular fibrillation, the myocardium is depolarizing at random, resulting in uncoordinated electrical activity, with subsequent loss of cardiac output and cardiac arrest. It is uncommon in infants and children, and causes include congenital heart disease, cardiomyopathy, electrolyte imbalance, hypothermia, drug toxicity and metabolic abnormalities (American Heart Association, 2000).

The ECG trace is very characteristic with bizarre and chaotic waveforms. Initially coarse (Fig. 7.1), the VF amplitude and waveform deteriorate

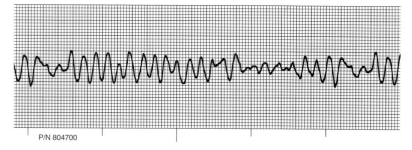

Fig. 7.1   Ventricular fibrillation (coarse).

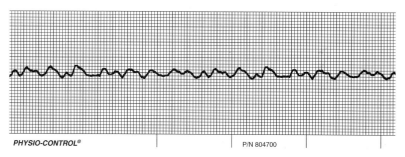

Fig. 7.2   Ventricular fibrillation (fine).

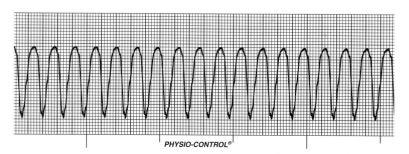

Fig. 7.3   Ventricular tachycardia.

rapidly, reflecting the depletion of myocardial high-energy phosphate stores (Mapin *et al.*, 1991) with fine VF developing (Fig. 7.2).

Early defibrillation is the definitive treatment; the chances of success decline substantially (7–10%) with each passing minute that there is a delay to defibrillation (Cobbe *et al.*, 1991). There is a slower decline if there is adequate BLS (Larsen *et al.*, 1993).

Pulseless ventricular tachycardia (Fig. 7.3) is treated in the same way as ventricular fibrillation.

Physiology of defibrillation

The heart can respond to an extrinsic electrical impulse just as it can respond to an impulse from the SA node or from an ectopic focus. It is thought that successful defibrillation occurs when a critical mass of myocardium is depolarized by the passage of an electric current (Resuscitation Council (UK), 2000a).

If a critical mass (75–90%) of cells are in the same phase (recovery or repolarization) when the current is removed, defibrillation occurs and the SA node or another intrinsic pacemaker can then regain control (Zhou *et al.*, 1980).

Success will depend on the actual current flow rather than shock energy. This current flow is influenced by transthoracic impedance (resistance of the chest tissues), electrode position and shock energy delivered. Only a small proportion of the energy delivered actually reaches the myocardium (Lermann and Deale, 1990); an effective technique is essential to optimize the chances of successful defibrillation.

Factors affecting successful defibrillation

As well as early delivery following the onset of VF, there are a number of factors that can influence the likelihood of successful defibrillation. These are discussed below.

Shock energy

Energy levels set too low will fail to defibrillate a critical mass of the myocardium, while those set too high may damage the myocardium and surrounding tissues. If VF fails to respond to the first shock, it is highly likely to respond to the second shock of the same energy, partly because transthoracic impedance is reduced (Resuscitation Council (UK), 2000a). Selecting the appropriate energy levels reduces the number of repetitive shocks and limits myocardial damage (Joglar *et al.*, 1999).

The optimum shock energy for defibrillation in infants and children has yet to be determined (American Academy of Pediatrics, 1997). The recommended initial shock energy levels are 2 J/kg followed by 2 J/kg. If these shocks fail, 4 J/kg is then advocated for all subsequent shocks required during the CPR attempt. If defibrillation is transiently successful and there is a return of cardiac output, but the patient subsequently reverts back to VF, shock energy levels revert back to 2 J/kg. If biphasic waveform shocks are used, lower energy levels will be used.

Transthoracic impedance

If defibrillation is to be successful, sufficient electrical current needs to pass through the chest and depolarize a critical mass of myocardium. Transthoracic impedance is the resistance to the flow of current through the chest; the greater the resistance, the less the current flow. There are several factors that can influence transthoracic impedance, and correct defibrillation technique is essential to minimize their effect and maximize current flow to the myocardium.

Paddle size   The larger the paddles, the lower the transthoracic imped-ance (Connell *et al.*, 1973). Paddle size selection is based on providing the largest surface area of paddle contact with the chest wall without contact between the paddles (American Heart Association, 2000). Adult-sized paddles (8–10 cm in diameter) are generally suitable in children >1 year of age. Although paediatric paddles (Fig. 7.4) are associated with high transthoracic impedance (Atkins *et al.*, 1988a), for practical reasons they are generally recommended in infants <10 kg (approximately <12 months

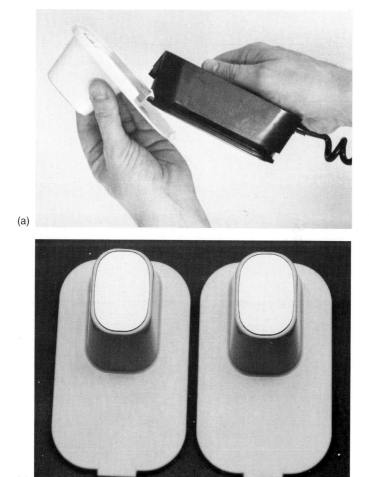

(a)

(b)

Fig. 7.4   Paediatric defibrillation paddles.

old) (Atkins and Kerber, 1992). If paediatric paddles are not available and defibrillation is required in an infant, adult paddles can be used, but positioned in the anteroposterior position (ALSG, 2001).

Paddle–skin interface If no paddle–skin interface is used, there will be high transthoracic impedance (Sirna *et al.*, 1988). Defibrillation gel pads (Fig. 7.5) should be used to reduce the impedance between the paddles and the skin (they can also help prevent skin burns). Defibrillation gel is now rarely used. It can be messy and any 'stray' gel can lead to arcing on the chest. Defibrillation gel pads are far superior.

Paddle pressure Pressing the paddles down firmly to the chest wall will help ensure good contact and reduce transthoracic impedance (Kerber *et al.*, 1981).

Time interval between shocks When shocks are delivered in close sequence, each will reduce transthoracic impedance for the following shock (Sirna *et al.*, 1988).

Phase of ventilation Air is a poor conductor of electricity. There is reduced impedance when shocks are delivered at the end of full expiration compared to inspiration (Sirna *et al.*, 1988).

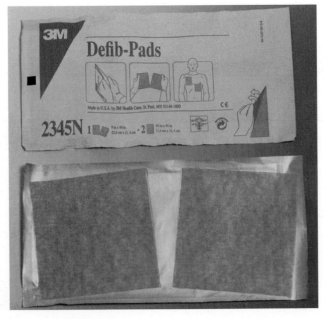

Fig. 7.5 Defibrillation gel pads.

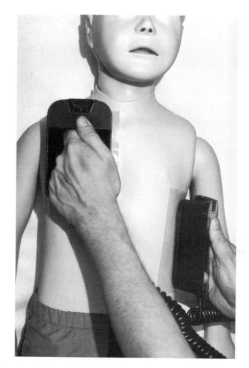

Fig. 7.6   Standard paddle position for defibrillation.

Paddle (electrode) position   The paddles should be placed to maximize the current flow through the myocardium. The polarity of the paddles is unimportant for defibrillation (Bardy *et al.*, 1989), though for ECG monitoring and cardioversion they should be placed according to their namesakes (sternum and apex).

The most commonly used paddle position is one paddle on the anterior chest, just to the right of the sternum (not over the sternum) below the right clavicle and the other on the lower left chest, to the left of the nipple (American Heart Association, 2000) (Fig. 7.6). The anteroposterior paddle position, although theoretically superior, is not practical in the emergency situation. However, it may be required if an infant requires defibrillation and only adult-sized paddles are available (American Academy of Pediatrics, 1997).

Safety issues and defibrillation

There are a number of safety issues related to defibrillation. It is important to:

- Diagnose cardiac arrest and ascertain that the ECG trace displays a shockable rhythm.

- Apply defibrillation gel pads to the child's bare chest to minimize the risk of skin burns (plus improve conduction).
- Avoid direct and indirect contact with the child (Gibbs *et al.*, 1990). All personnel should be well away from the bed and not touching the child or anything attached to the patient/bed, e.g. i.v. infusion stands, i.v. infusions. Be wary of wet surroundings.
- Temporarily remove oxygen away from the child (unless there is a closed circuit, i.e. the patient is intubated).
- Apply adequate pressure to the paddles to help minimize the risk of arcing.
- Charge the paddles either on the child's chest (preferable) or on the defibrillator in their allocated storage site.
- Shout 'stand clear' and check that all personnel are safely clear prior to defibrillation.
- Check the ECG monitor immediately prior to defibrillation; sometimes the ECG can revert to a non-shockable rhythm.
- Ask a colleague to increase the energy level on the defibrillator when required. If the practitioner is alone, return one paddle to the defibrillator and use the free hand to increase the energy level.

Procedure for manual defibrillation

The following procedure for manual defibrillation is based on Resuscitation Council (UK) (2000a) recommendations:

1. Confirm cardiac arrest and ensure that the cardiac arrest team or similar are alerted.
2. Ascertain that the ECG rhythm is VF/VT.
3. Place defibrillation gel pads on the child's bare chest, one just to the right of the sternum, below the right clavicle, and the other on the lower left chest, to the left of the nipple in the anterior axillary line.
4. Select 2 J/kg on the defibrillator. For defibrillators with stepped current levels the nearest higher step to the calculated level of joules should be selected (Zideman and Spearpoint, 1999).
5. Apply the defibrillator paddles firmly on the defibrillation pads.
6. Press the charge button on the paddles to charge the defibrillator and shout 'stand clear'.
7. Perform a visual check of the area to ensure that all personnel are clear.
8. Check the monitor to ensure that the child is still in VF/VT.
9. Press both discharge buttons simultaneously to discharge the shock.
10. Leaving the defibrillator paddles on the child's chest, wait for a few seconds before reassessing the ECG trace (this will allow it to stabilize). If VF/VT is confirmed, repeat steps 5–9. If uncertain about the ECG or if the ECG displayed is compatible with a cardiac output, recheck the pulse.
11. Return paddles to the defibrillator if shock not required.

Points to note

- Safety precautions should be observed.
- The paddles should remain on the child's chest between shocks, to minimize delays in defibrillation.
- Pulse checks following defibrillation are only recommended if an ECG compatible with a cardiac output is produced or if there is uncertainty regarding accurate interpretation of the ECG.
- BLS should not interrupt the sequence of shocks unless there are undue delays with defibrillation.
- If monitoring through the paddles, spurious asystole may be displayed following the delivery of a shock (Bradbury *et al.*, 2000). Monitoring using ECG leads is recommended to confirm the rhythm.
- If biphasic waveform shocks are used, lower energy levels will be required.

Automated external defibrillation

Operating a manual defibrillator requires extensive training and knowledge. Its use has therefore been traditionally restricted to doctors, and senior nurses working in critical care areas. However, the modern automated external defibrillator (AED) provides spoken and/or visual prompts and abolishes the need for the operator to have ECG interpretation skills. AEDs are commonly used in the management of adult cardiac arrests, particularly in the prehospital situation.

The use of AEDs in children is extremely limited. Although they can accurately identify VF in children of all ages (Atkins *et al.*, 1998b; Cecchin *et al.*, 1999), there have been concerns regarding inadequate data on their accuracy in correctly identifying tachycardic rhythms in infants (Hazinski *et al.*, 1997). In addition, the use of AEDs with adult fixed-rate energy levels in children <8 years is not advocated (American Heart Association, 2000).

However, AEDs intended for use in children <8 years are currently being developed and evaluated. One manufacturer now has FDA approval for the use of its AED with paediatric pads, which will deliver a fixed rate of 50 J. When using the specially designed paediatric pads (Fig. 7.7), the AED can be used on infants and children <8 years of age. The pads are applied in the anteroposterior position.

The following procedure for the use of the FR2 with the paediatric pads is based on the manufacturer's recommendations:

1. Switch on the AED and follow spoken and/or visual prompts.
2. Ensure that the child's skin is dry.
3. Attach the defibrillation electrodes: one on the chest and one on the back.
4. Stand clear while the AED performs ECG analysis. Ensure nobody touches the child during ECG analysis. This is to prevent artefactual errors during ECG analysis. In addition, patient movement can interrupt and delay ECG analysis.

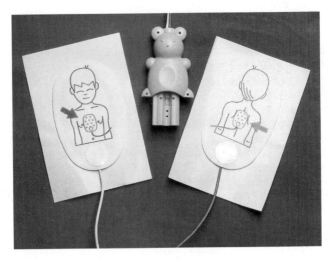

Fig. 7.7   Paediatric automated external defibrillation pads.

5. If shock is advised, shout 'stand clear' and perform visual check to ensure that all staff are clear. The AED will automatically charge to 50 J.
6. Ensure that all personnel are clear of the patient and press the shock button as indicated.
7. Repeat step 4 and then steps 5 and 6 if necessary.
8. After three shocks, or if no shock is advised, check for signs of circulation. If there are no signs of circulation, perform CPR for 1 minute. The AED will reanalyse after 1 minute.

Procedure for synchronized cardioversion

Synchronized cardioversion is a reliable method of converting a tachyarrhythmia to sinus rhythm (Resuscitation Council (UK), 2000a). Owing to the associated risks, it is generally only undertaken when pharmacological intervention has been unsuccessful or if the child is haemodynamically compromised.

The shock should be delivered on the R wave and not on the vulnerable T wave – synchronizing the delivered energy with the ECG will reduce the risk of inducing ventricular fibrillation (Lown, 1967). This is accomplished by securing a reliable ECG trace (usually lead II) using the defibrillator monitor and by pressing the 'synchronized' button on the defibrillator. A dot or arrow should only appear on the R waves.

The following procedure for emergency cardioversion is based on Resuscitation Council (UK) (2000a) recommendations:

1. Attach ECG leads and establish an accurate ECG trace. Lead II is usually selected. The defibrillator should be used for cardiac monitoring, otherwise synchronization will not be possible.

2. Activate the 'synchronized' button on the defibrillator.
3. Check that only the R waves are being synchronized; a dot or an arrow should appear on each R wave and not on other parts of the ECG complex, e.g. tall T waves.
4. Place defibrillation gel pads on the child's chest (see p. 83).
5. Select the required energy dose – 0.5–1 J/kg (this is increased to 2 J/kg for subsequent shocks) (ALSG, 2001).
6. Apply the defibrillator paddles firmly on the defibrillation pads. It is important to apply the paddles according to their namesakes, i.e. sternum to sternum and apex to apex.
7. Press the charge button on the paddles to charge the defibrillator and shout 'stand clear'.
8. Perform a visual check of the area to ensure that all personnel are clear.
9. Check the monitor to ensure that the child is still in the tachyarrhythmia that requires synchronized cardioversion. Also check that the synchronized button is still activated and is synchronizing on only the R waves.
10. Press both discharge buttons simultaneously to discharge the shock. There will be a slight delay (until the next R wave) between pressing the shock buttons and shock discharge.

Points to note

• Consent of the child's parents or carers should be obtained if possible.
• CPR equipment should be immediately available in case of cardiac arrest following the procedure.
• A conscious child will need to be sedated or anaesthetized – ideally an anaesthetist should be present.
• Following cardioversion, the 'synch' button will usually need to be reactivated if further cardioversion is required. However, on some defibrillators the 'synch' button will remain activated once pressed and therefore needs to be switched off once no further cardioversion is required.
• Antiarrhythmic therapy may be required if initial cardioversion attempts are unsuccessful.

Summary

The ECG characteristics and pathophysiology of VF have been described. The factors affecting successful defibrillation, together with safety issues have been discussed. The procedures for manual defibrillation, automated external defibrillation and emergency synchronized cardioversion have been described. If indicated, defibrillation should be performed rapidly, safely and effectively.

Chapter 8

Advanced life support

Introduction

Paediatric advanced life support (PALS) is the term used to describe the more specialized techniques employed to support breathing and circulation during paediatric CPR, as well as specific treatment used to try to restore cardiac output.

The European Resuscitation Council PALS algorithm (2001) (Fig. 8.1) is universally applicable, though specific modifications are required to maximize the likelihood of success in some special situations (Chs 9 and 10).

The aim of this chapter is to understand the principles of the European Resuscitation Council Paediatric ALS guidelines.

Objectives

At the end of the chapter the reader will be able to:

• outline the European Resuscitation Council PALS algorithm
• outline the principles of intraosseous infusion
• discuss the tracheal route for drug administration
• discuss the use of resuscitation drugs
• discuss the treatment of potentially reversible causes of paediatric cardiac arrest
• outline the treatment of bradyarrhythmias and tachyarrhythmias.

European Resuscitation Council PALS algorithm

The European Resuscitation Council PALS algorithm (Fig. 8.1) is designed to be an aide-memoire, reminding the practitioner of the important aspects of assessment and treatment of a paediatric cardiac arrest. It is not designed to be comprehensive or limiting. Each step that follows in the algorithm assumes that the previous one has been unsuccessful. Looping the algorithm reinforces the concept of constant assessment and reassessment.

BLS algorithm: ventilate/oxygenate

PALS initially involves the establishment of effective basic life support and ventilation (Zideman and Spearpoint, 1999). The airway should be opened and positive pressure ventilation with a high inspired oxygen concentration should be provided. In some situations these interventions may be all that is required to resuscitate the child (Bingham, 1996).

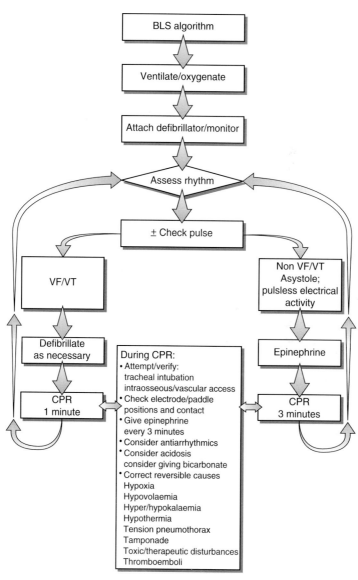

Fig. 8.1 European Resuscitation Council paediatric advanced life support algorithm 2001 (reproduced with permission of Aurum Pharmaceuticals).

Attach defibrillator/monitor

As soon as the defibrillator/monitor arrives, ECG monitoring should be established (Ch. 6). Select lead II on the monitor and attach the ECG leads as follows:

- *red* on the right shoulder
- *yellow* on the left shoulder
- *green* on the left upper abdominal wall.

Another option is to monitor the ECG using the defibrillator paddles. Select 'Paddles' setting on the defibrillator and apply gel pads and paddles to chest (see Fig. 7.6, p. 83).

Assess rhythm

The presenting cardiac arrest arrhythmia can then be classified into one of two groups, dependent upon whether defibrillation is required (VF/VT) or is not required (non-VF/VT). The appropriate pathway in the algorithm can then be followed.

If ECG monitoring has already been established prior to the arrest, the presenting cardiac arrest arrhythmia can be assessed immediately to ascertain which loop of the algorithm to follow.

VF/VT pathway

If VF/VT (Fig. 8.2) is identified (rare), defibrillation should be performed as soon as possible (a precordial thump may be delivered if the child is monitored, if the onset of VF/VT is witnessed and if the defibrillator is not immediately at hand (ALSG, 2001)).

The recommended initial energy sequence for defibrillatory shocks is:

- 2 J/kg
- 2 J/kg
- 4 J/kg

(or biphasic equivalent).

If the first 2 J/kg fails, the second 2 J/kg may be successful if delivered promptly because of reduced tissue impedance. All subsequent shocks

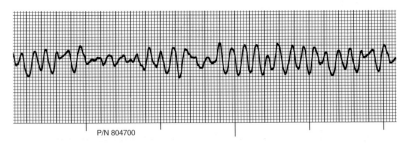

P/N 804700

Fig. 8.2 Ventricular fibrillation.

should be at 4 J/kg (if, after a return of spontaneous circulation, VF/VT recurs, restart at 2 J/kg again).

After each shock the ECG is reassessed to ascertain whether further defibrillation is required. Pulse checks following defibrillation are only recommended if an ECG compatible with a cardiac output is produced (including ventricular tachycardia) or if there is uncertainty regarding the interpretation of the ECG. BLS should not interrupt the sequence of shocks unless there are undue delays with defibrillation. If three shocks are required, the aim is to deliver them within 1 minute.

If the first three shocks are unsuccessful, the priority changes to the provision of BLS (5 compressions : 1 ventilation, or asynchronous if the child is intubated) for 1 minute to help preserve cerebral and myocardial function. During this time the child should be intubated. Intravenous or intraosseous access should be secured and epinephrine (adrenaline) 10 µg/kg (0.1 ml/kg of 1 : 10 000 solution) administered. If venous access has not been secured, epinephrine (adrenaline) can be administered down the tracheal tube at a dose of 100 µg/kg (1 ml/kg of 1 : 10 000 solution or 0.1 ml/kg 1 : 1000 solution).

After 1 minute of BLS, the ECG trace is reassessed and a further sequence of up to three shocks of 4 J/kg delivered if required. Each loop of the algorithm provides a further opportunity, if not already done, to secure venous access and attempt tracheal intubation. The accuracy of the ECG trace should be regularly verified. Epinephrine (adrenaline) is administered every 3 minutes.

In refractory VF, an antiarrhythmic, e.g. amiodarone, should be considered, as well as a different defibrillator and an alternative paddle position (ALSG, 2001). Any reversible causes, e.g. hypothermia and electrolyte imbalance, should be treated. An alkalizing agent should be considered in a prolonged arrest.

Non-VF/VT pathway

If VF/VT can be positively excluded, defibrillation is not indicated at this stage and the non-VF/VT pathway of the algorithm should be followed. The main arrhythmias normally seen are either asystole or pulseless electrical activity (PEA), formally known as electromechanical dissociation or EMD.

Asystole (Fig. 8.3) is the most common cardiac arrest arrhythmia in children (ALSG, 2001). Great care should be taken to ensure that the ECG trace is accurate and that the 'straight line' is not due to a mechanical problem. Check the:

• ECG leads are correctly attached
• correct monitoring lead has been selected (normally lead II)
• ECG gain (ECG size).

Asystole is rarely a straight line. Spurious asystole may be displayed following defibrillation if monitoring through defibrillation paddles – the

ECG trace should be confirmed by monitoring through ECG leads (Bradbury *et al.*, 2000). It is most important that a potentially treatable rhythm, e.g. ventricular fibrillation, is not missed. Cardiac pacing is ineffective in the management of asystole (Quan *et al.*, 1992).

PEA is a clinical condition of cardiac arrest, but in the presence of a normal or near normal ECG trace (Fig. 8.4). It can be either primary or secondary. Primary PEA results from the failure of the myocardium to respond to electrical stimulation, e.g. in hypoxia (Skinner and Vincent, 1997); secondary PEA occurs where mechanical barriers to ventricular filling or cardiac output are present, e.g. tension pneumothorax (Colquhoun and Camm, 1999). The child's optimal chance for survival rests with the prompt identification and treatment of any underlying cause (see below).

If asystole or PEA is confirmed, BLS (5 compressions:1 ventilation, or asynchronous if the child is intubated) is undertaken for 3 minutes. During this time the child should be intubated. Intravenous or intraosseous access should be secured and epinephrine (adrenaline) 10 μg/kg (0.1 ml/kg of 1:10 000 solution) administered. If venous access has not been secured, adrenaline (epinephrine) can be administered down the tracheal tube at a dose of 100 μg/kg (1 ml/kg of 1:10 000 solution or 0.1 ml/kg 1:1000 solution).

After 3 minutes of CPR the ECG trace should be reassessed and the appropriate pathway followed. Epinephrine (adrenaline) is repeated every

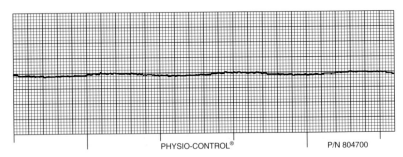

Fig. 8.3 Asystole.

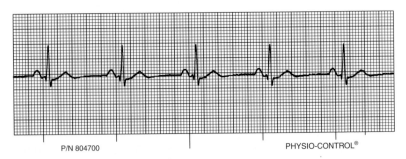

Fig. 8.4 Pulseless electrical activity (PEA).

3 minutes and, if the cause of the cardiac arrest is circulatory collapse or if continuous intra-arterial monitoring is available, higher doses may be administered (ALSG, 2001). Other medications, e.g. alkalizing agents, should be considered and potentially reversible causes should be treated (see below). The accuracy of the ECG trace should be regularly verified. Any reversible causes should be treated.

Principles of intraosseous infusion

Establishing vascular access is crucial for drug and fluid administration. However, obtaining i.v. access in a paediatric arrest is notoriously difficult (Zideman and Spearpoint, 1999) and any delays in securing it may compromise the resuscitation attempt (Rosetti *et al.*, 1984, 1985). It is therefore recommended to try the intraosseous route first if there is no circulatory access in place (ALSG, 2001; European Resuscitation Council, 2001).

Intraosseous infusion is a quick, reliable and relatively easy method of establishing vascular access. It can be used for the administration of drugs, fluids and blood products in infants and small children in the resuscitation situation (Berg, 1984; Glaeser and Losek, 1986; McNamara *et al.*, 1987). A selection of intraosseous needles is available (Fig. 8.5).

Advantages of intraosseous infusion include:

• quick to establish – in the majority of cases within 30–60 seconds, even by practitioners with limited experience (Glaeser *et al.*, 1988; Seigler *et al.*, 1989)
• onset of action and drug levels are comparable with conventional intravenous access (Andropoulos *et al.*, 1990)
• blood sampling for laboratory studies is possible (Johnson *et al.*, 1999).

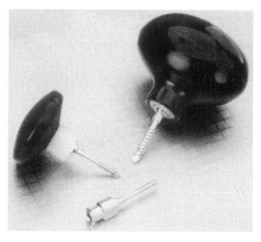

Fig. 8.5 Intraosseous needle (Cook Incorporated, Bloomington, IN, USA).

Procedure for intraosseous infusion

1. Locate the site of access – the most commonly used site is on the antero-medial surface of the tibia, 2–3 cm below the tibial tuberosity (ALSG, 2001). There is a large bone marrow cavity here and minimal risk to adjacent tissues. This is the preferred site in children <6 years of age (American Academy of Pediatrics, 1997).
2. Clean with antiseptic solution (if circumstances permit).
3. Check that the outer needle and internal stylet of the intraosseous needle are properly aligned.
4. Stabilize the child's leg. Using the palm of the non-dominant hand, grasp the thigh and knee above and lateral to the insertion site, and wrap the thumb and fingers around the knee (American Academy of Pediatrics, 1997). It is important to ensure that no part of your hand is allowed to rest behind the insertion site (under the leg).
5. Insert the needle into the bone at right-angles to the long axis of the bone, in a slight caudal direction to avoid the epiphysial plate. Adopt a gentle but firm twisting or drilling technique (American Academy of Pediatrics, 1997) (Fig. 8.6). As it passes through the bony cortex into the marrow, a sudden drop in resistance should be felt. If the needle is in the correct position:
   - it should stay upright without support
   - it should be possible to aspirate bone marrow
   - fluid can be injected through the needle, without evidence of it infil-trating the surrounding tissues.
6. Once successful insertion has been confirmed, flush the cannula, secure it with tape and connect a primed infusion tubing with a three-way tap.

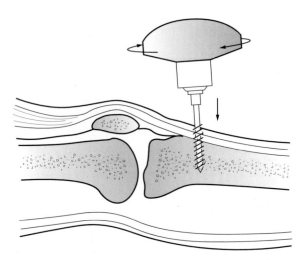

Fig. 8.6   Intraosseous needle insertion (Cook Incorporated, Bloomington, IN, USA).

7. Send a bone marrow sample for laboratory studies (inform the technician that it is bone marrow to avoid unnecessary damage to laboratory equipment).
8. Use a 20-ml syringe to inject fluids and medications (ALSG, 2001). This is necessary to overcome resistance.
9. Flush with normal saline to ensure that medications are delivered to the central circulation (American Academy of Pediatrics, 1997).

Complications of intraosseous infusion are low (Heinild *et al.*, 1974; Rosetti *et al.*, 1985) and the long-term effects of intraosseous infusion on the bone marrow and bone growth are minimal (Fiser *et al.*, 1997). However, the following complications have been reported:

- fractured tibia (La Fleche *et al.*, 1989)
- lower extremity compartment syndrome (Vidal *et al.*, 1993)
- severe extravasion of medications (Simmons *et al.*, 1994)
- osteomyelitis (Rosovsky *et al.*, 1994).

Although complications are rare, they can be severe. Consequently, intraosseous infusion should only be undertaken in critically ill infants and children (as a temporary measure until other venous access sites have been secured) (Fuchs *et al.*, 1991).

Tracheal route for drug administration

Both clinical and experimental studies have reported conflicting evidence about the efficacy of the tracheal tube route for drug administration (Jevon, 2002). It is therefore only recommended as a second-line approach (if i.v. or intraosseous access is not available) (ALSG, 2001). The following drugs can be administered via this route (Johnston, 1992) and can be remembered by the mnemonic LEAN:

- *L*idocaine (lignocaine)
- *E*pinephrine (adrenaline)
- *A*tropine
- *N*aloxone.

When using the tracheal route for drug administration, higher drug doses are recommended (American Heart Association, 2000), e.g. epinephrine (adrenaline): 0.1 mg/kg (0.1 ml/kg of 1:1000 solution), i.e. 10 times the standard i.v. dose. It is suggested to dilute the drug in up to 5 ml of normal saline and follow the administration with five manual ventilations (Jasani *et al.*, 1994). The rate of absorption will depend on the efficiency of CPR and will be reduced if pulmonary oedema is present (Jevon, 2002).

Resuscitation drugs

Epinephrine (adrenaline)

Epinephrine (Fig. 8.7a) is administered routinely in most resuscitation attempts every 3–5 minutes. It improves coronary and cerebral blood flow

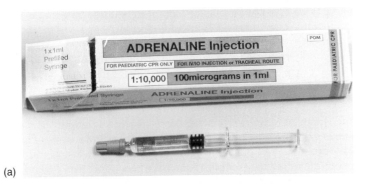

(a)

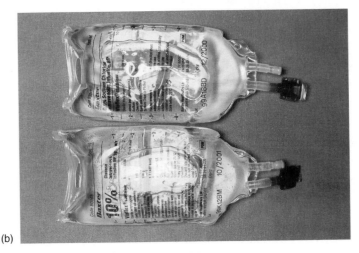

(b)

Fig. 8.7 Resuscitation drugs (a) and fluids (b).

(Schleien *et al.*, 1986). It also increases the vigour and intensity of VF, which may contribute to successful defibrillation (Otto *et al.*, 1981). Because acidosis and hypoxaemia can depress the action of epinephrine (adrenaline) (Huang *et al.*, 1995), it is important to ensure that effective ventilations and chest compressions are continued.

The recommended dose is $10\,\mu g/kg$ ($0.1\,ml/kg$ of $1:10\,000$ solution), repeated every 3–5 minutes for ongoing arrest (American Heart Association, 2000). If the tracheal route is used, $100\,\mu g/kg$ ($0.1\,ml/kg$ of $1:1000$ solution) is recommended. However, the resulting plasma concentrations are unpredictable (Kleinman *et al.*, 1999).

A higher dose ($100\,\mu g/kg$) may also be considered if the cause of the arrest was extreme vasodilatation, e.g. in septicaemia and anaphylaxis, or if an arterial pressure monitoring is already in place (i.e. the effect can be monitored) (Resuscitation Council (UK), 2000c).

Atropine

The most likely cause of bradycardia in infants and children is hypoxia. Initial treatment therefore involves ensuring adequate ventilation and oxygenation and if drug therapy is required, epinephrine (adrenaline) is usually administered (American Heart Association, 2000).

Atropine is sometimes administered for symptomatic bradyarrhythmias, particularly if induced by vagal stimulation during suction or tracheal intubation (ALSG, 2001). If administered, the recommended dose of atropine is 20 μg/kg i.v. As small doses of atropine can cause paradoxical bradycardia, a minimum dose of 100 μg is recommended (Dauchot and Gravenstein, 1971). It can be administered via the tracheal route (Howard and Bingham, 1990), though the absorption into the circulation is unpredictable (Lee *et al.*, 1989).

Amiodarone

Amiodarone should be considered in refractory VF/VT (i.e. when the first three defibrillatory shocks have been unsuccessful). The recommended dose is 5 mg/kg administered by a rapid i.v. bolus followed by BLS and further defibrillation within 1 minute (ALSG, 2001).

Lidocaine (lignocaine)

Lidocaine (lignocaine) is usually only used when amiodarone is not available. It should then be considered in refractory VF/VT (i.e. when the first three defibrillatory shocks have been unsuccessful). The recommended dose is 1 mg/kg administered by a rapid i.v. bolus.

Calcium

The routine use of calcium does not improve the outcome from cardiac arrest (Stueven *et al.*, 1985a,b). It may have detrimental effects in the ischaemic myocardium and may impair cerebral recovery (Resuscitation Council (UK), 2000a). Specific indications for its use include:

- hypocalcaemia – relatively common in critically ill children (American Heart Association, 2000), particularly in septicaemia (Cardenas-Rivero *et al.*, 1989)
- hyperkalaemia (Bisogno *et al.*, 1994)
- hypermagnesaemia (ALSG, 2001)
- calcium channel blocker overdose.

The dose is 0.2 ml/kg of 10% calcium chloride i.v. Careful administration is required as extravasation around the cannula may cause severe tissue injury. It should not be administered simultaneously with sodium bicarbonate via the same route. The tracheal route should not be used.

Sodium bicarbonate

Although sodium bicarbonate has been traditionally administered for the treatment of severe metabolic acidosis associated with cardiac arrest, it has not been shown to improve outcome (Levy, 1998). In addition there are numerous detrimental side-effects including:

- generation of carbon dioxide
- exacerbation of intracellular acidosis
- impaired oxygen delivery to the tissues (Bellingham *et al.*, 1971)
- metabolic alkalosis
- hypernatraemia (Aufderheide *et al.*, 1992)
- hyperosmolality (Bishop and Weisfeltd, 1976).

Respiratory failure is the major cause of cardiac arrest in children. As sodium bicarbonate raises carbon dioxide tension, its administration in a paediatric arrest may in fact worsen existing respiratory acidosis (American Heart Association, 2000). Consequently, the initial priority in paediatric resuscitation is attention to ABC.

Indications for considering administering sodium bicarbonate include:

- prolonged cardiac arrest – usually considered if spontaneous circulation has not returned following the first or second dose of adrenaline (epinephrine) (ALSG, 2001)
- shock associated with documented metabolic acidosis (American Heart Association, 2000)
- hyperkalaemia (Ettinger *et al.*, 1974)
- tricyclic overdose (Hoffman *et al.*, 1993).

If administered, the recommended dose is 1 mmol/kg (1 ml/kg of 8.4% solution) (ALSG, 2001). A flush with 0.9% sodium chloride should always precede and follow administration (it can inactivate other drugs). Care should be taken, as extravasion may cause severe tissue injury. The tracheal route should not be used.

Adequate ventilation must be maintained to avoid respiratory acidosis (the bicarbonate ion is excreted as carbon dioxide via the lungs). The blood pH and base excess should also be monitored, though the accuracy of arterial blood gas analysis during cardiac arrest or severe shock has been questioned (Weil *et al.*, 1986; Steedman and Robertson, 1992).

Magnesium

Indications for administering magnesium include:

- hypomagnesaemia
- torsades de pointes VT (Banai and Tzivoni, 1993).

The recommended dose is 25–50 mg/kg (max. 2 g) in a rapid i.v. infusion over several minutes (ALSG, 2001).

Fluids

If the cardiac arrest has resulted from circulatory failure, a standard bolus of crystalloid fluid, e.g. 0.9% sodium chloride (Fig. 8.7b), should be administered if there is no response to the first dose of epinephrine (adrenaline)

(ALSG, 2001). The recommended volume is 20 ml/kg (American Heart Association, 2000).

Blood administration is recommended in children with severe haemorrhage who have not responded to 40–60 ml/kg of crystalloid (American Heart Association, 2000).

(Although the use of colloid solutions in adult resuscitation may be associated with increased mortality (Schierhout and Roberts, 1998), there are insufficient data at present to advise against their use in children (American Heart Association, 2000).)

Glucose

Infants and children have high glucose requirements (particularly when seriously ill) and low glycogen stores. However, it is not known whether the administration of glucose improves cardiac function and survival of hypoglycaemic children in cardiac arrest (American Academy of Pediatrics, 1997). In fact the administration of glucose during resuscitation may be associated with a worse outcome (D'Alecy *et al.*, 1986; Nakakimura *et al.*, 1990).

The routine use of glucose in resuscitation is therefore not recommended, except when documented hypoglycaemia is present (American Academy of Pediatrics, 1997). If glucose is required, the recommended dose is 0.5 g/kg dextrose (5 ml/kg of 10% dextrose) (ALSG, 2001) (Fig. 8.7b).

Hyperglycaemia should be avoided as it will increase cerebral metabolism (Oakley and Redmond, 1999) and may have detrimental effects on neurological outcome (Pulsineli *et al.*, 1982; Sieber and Traystman, 1992; Cherian *et al.*, 1997). In addition, hyperglycaemia will cause a sharp rise in serum osmolality, which may result in osmotic diuresis (American Heart Association, 2000).

Potentially reversible causes of cardiac arrest

As it is rare for infants and children to have a primary cardiac arrest, it is important to identify and treat the initial cause of the cardiorespiratory collapse (Zideman and Spearpoint, 1999). The search for, and treatment of, potentially reversible causes of cardiac arrest is paramount, particularly when PEA is present. These causes can conveniently be classified into two groups for ease of memory – four 'Hs' and four 'Ts'.

- *H*ypoxia
- *H*ypovolaemia
- *H*yperkalaemia/hypokalaemia
- *H*ypothermia
- *T*ension pneumothorax
- *T*amponade
- *T*oxic/therapeutic disturbances
- *T*hromboemboli.

If the underlying cause is detected, it should be treated rapidly and appropriately (Zideman and Spearpoint, 1999). The treatment of these causes is now briefly discussed.

Hypoxia

The airway should be secured and ventilation with 100% oxygen continued.

Hypovolaemia

Causes could include severe haemorrhage and severe diarrhoea and vomiting; intravascular volume should be restored using appropriate fluids, plus urgent surgical referral arranged if haemorrhage is suspected.

Hyperkalaemia/hypokalaemia

The diagnosis can be confirmed by laboratory tests, though the child's history, e.g. renal disease, may be suggestive of abnormal blood chemistry. If possible, the disorder should be corrected. Calcium is usually administered if hyperkalaemia is suspected or confirmed (Bisogno *et al.*, 1994).

Hypothermia

This should be particularly suspected following an immersion injury. A low-reading thermometer should be used and if necessary the child should be rapidly rewarmed (see pp. 111–112).

Tension pneumothorax

Causes include chest trauma, asthma and central venous cannulation. A needle thoracocentesis is usually performed initially (second intercostal space, midclavicular line, on the affected side) and followed by the insertion of a chest drain.

Tamponade

Tamponade occurs when blood or other fluid fills the pericardial space, raising intrapericardial pressure, compressing the heart and preventing it from filling. Clinical features include distended neck veins, hypotension and muffled heart sounds. Unfortunately these can be obscured by the cardiac arrest itself. It can occur following both blunt and penetrating trauma (ALSG, 2001). Initially a needle pericardiocentesis is performed to relieve the tamponade.

Toxic/therapeutic disturbances

If there is no specific history related to toxic or therapeutic disturbances, the cause may only be established following laboratory investigations. If applicable, the appropriate antidote should be administered. Treatment is often only supportive.

Thromboemboli

Although very rare, if a pulmonary embolism is suspected, an emergency pulmonary embolectomy may be required. If possible, the child should be transferred to a cardiovascular surgical department.

Treatment of bradyarrhythmias and tachyarrhythmias

Bradyarrhythmias

The majority of bradyarrhythmias are secondary to hypoxia and shock and are pre-terminal events (ALSG, 2001). Bradycardia that is clinically significant can be defined as a heart rate < 60 or a rapidly falling heart rate despite adequate oxygenation and ventilation, associated with poor systemic perfusion (American Academy of Pediatrics, 2000). Causes of bradyarrhythmias include hypoxia, acidosis, hypothermia and excessive vagal stimulation.

As the most likely cause of bradycardia in infants and children is hypoxia, the initial treatment involves ensuring adequate ventilation and oxygenation. If present, circulatory shock should also be treated with volume expansion (American Heart Association, 2000). If these measures are ineffective, epinephrine (adrenaline) 10 μg/kg i.v. bolus, followed by an infusion, should be considered (ALSG, 2001).

Atropine is sometimes administered for symptomatic bradyarrhythmias, particularly if induced by vagal stimulation during suction or tracheal intubation (ALSG, 2001). If administered, the recommended dose of atropine is 20 μg/kg i.v. As small doses of atropine can cause paradoxical bradycardia, a minimum dose of 100 μg is recommended (Dauchot and Gravenstein, 1971). Maximum doses of atropine are 1 mg in children and 2 mg in adolescents (American Heart Association, 2000).

Cardiac pacing can be life saving in rare situations, e.g. complete AV block or SA node malfunction (Beland *et al.*, 1987). However, it is not beneficial if the bradycardia is secondary to a post-arrest hypoxic/ischaemic myocardial insult or respiratory failure (Quan *et al.*, 1992).

Tachyarrhythmias

Supraventricular tachycardia is the most common non-arrest cardiac arrhythmia in children and the most common cardiac arrhythmia in infants that produces cardiovascular instability (ALSG, 2001). The ventricular rate in SVT is typically > 220. Ideally a 12-lead ECG should be recorded to help confirm diagnosis.

The child's age, ventricular rate, duration of SVT and ventricular function prior to the onset all influence the haemodynamic effect of SVT (American Heart Association, 2000). Treatment options for SVT include:

Vagal manoeuvres   Ice water applied to the face is the most effective method in infants and young children (Aydin *et al.*, 1995); carotid sinus massage appears to be safe and effective in older children (Lim *et al.*, 1998);

asking the child to blow through a straw is another method (Lim *et al.*, 1998).

Adenosine   This is the drug of choice (Losek *et al.*, 1999); the initial recommended dose is 100 µg/kg i.v. bolus, followed by a flush (Overholt *et al.*, 1988). ECG monitoring should continue during and after administration. It can be administered via the intraosseous route (Friedman, 1996).

Synchronized cardioversion   This is usually a last resort (see pp. 86–87).

Ventricular tachycardia is rare in childhood. If the child is pulseless, follow the PALS algorithm (VF/VT pathway). If the child has a pulse, administer oxygen, establish whether the child is haemodynamically compromised or not and if possible record a 12-lead ECG. Amiodarone 5 mg/kg i.v. over 20–60 minutes is usually administered (American Heart Association, 2000). If unstable, i.e. the child is severely compromised, synchronized cardioversion should be performed immediately (ALSG, 2001). Any electrolyte imbalances should be corrected.

NB: Ensure that expert help is called.

Summary

The European Resuscitation Council Paediatric ALS algorithm has been outlined. The principles of intraosseous infusion and the use of the tracheal route for drug administration have been described. The use of resuscitation drugs and the treatment of potentially reversible causes of paediatric cardiac arrest have been discussed. The treatment of bradyarrhythmias and tachyarrhythmias has been outlined.

Chapter 9

Anaphylaxis

Introduction

Anaphylaxis is an acute, severe, hypersensitivity reaction that can lead to asphyxia and cardiac arrest. Although the incidence is not known, it is thought to be on the increase, probably coinciding with a notable increase in the prevalence of allergic diseases in the last 30 years. It is often poorly managed; in particular epinephrine (adrenaline) is greatly under-used.

This has led to the publication of broad consensus guidelines by a Project Team of the Resuscitation Council (UK) (1999, 2001) on the appropriate emergency management of acute anaphylactic reactions by first medical responders. It must be stressed that these guidelines are not intended to replace existing advice for specific situations, e.g. specialist clinics (DoH, 1996).

The aim of this chapter is to understand the principles of the emergency management of anaphylaxis.

Objectives

At the end of the chapter the reader will be able to:

- define anaphylaxis
- discuss the pathophysiology of anaphylaxis
- list the causes of anaphylaxis
- describe the clinical features and diagnosis of anaphylaxis
- discuss the management of anaphylaxis.

Definition of anaphylaxis

Anaphylaxis is an exaggerated response of a previously sensitized individual to a drug or substance, typically mediated by immunoglobulin (IgE). Anaphylactoid reactions are similar but do not involve hypersensitivity. For this chapter, the term anaphylaxis will be used to describe both types of reactions because the initial treatment will be the same; only the follow-up care will differ.

Pathophysiology

When exposed to a specific antigen, antigen-specific immunoglobulin E (IgE) antibodies cause the release of histamine and vasoactive mediators from mast cells and basophils producing circulatory, respiratory, gastrointestinal and cutaneous effects. These effects can include the development of pharyngeal and laryngeal oedema, bronchospasm and decreased vascular tone and capillary leak causing circulatory collapse.

Causes

Exposure to the allergen can be through ingestion, injection, inhalation or skin contact (Wong *et al.*, 1999). Causes of anaphylaxis include:

- certain foods, e.g. shellfish, eggs and tomatoes; sometimes following just skin contact or inhalation (Tan *et al.*, 2001)
- peanuts and tree-borne nuts – particularly dangerous (Ewan, 1996)
- blood products
- immunizations
- bee/wasp stings
- contrast media (ALSG, 2001)
- drugs, e.g. penicillin
- latex, e.g. during surgery and from plastic balls in play pits (Fiocchi *et al.*, 2001)
- mites (Matsumoto *et al.*, 2001).

Clinical features and diagnosis

The clinical features will vary depending on the cause. For example:

- *ingested allergen* (e.g. peanut): usually lip, mucosal and laryngeal oedema together with bronchoconstriction (Clarke and Nasser, 2001)
- *injected or systemic allergens* (e.g. insect venom or contrast media): usually hypotension
- *allergen absorbed through the skin* (e.g. latex): slow onset as the allergen is absorbed through the skin (Ewan, 1998).

In addition, anaphylactic reactions can vary in severity and the process can be slow, rapid or biphasic; occasionally the onset may be delayed by up to 24 hours (Fisher, 1986). The more rapid the onset, the more severe is the reaction (Wong *et al.*, 1999). Clinical features could include:

- urticaria – usually the first presenting clinical feature (Morton and Phillips, 1992)
- tachycardia and hypotension
- pallor
- angio-oedema (facial swelling) – more noticeable in the eyelids, lips and tongue (Wong *et al.*, 1999)
- feeling of impending doom
- coughing/wheezing
- vomiting, abdominal pain and diarrhoea – particularly when caused by an ingested allergen (Morton and Phillips, 1996).

It is possible to mistake panic attack for anaphylaxis. A panic attack can lead to hyperventilation, an anxiety-related erythematous rash and tachycardia. However, there will be no hypotension, pallor, wheeze or urticarial rash.

The lack of a consistent clinical picture can sometimes make an accurate diagnosis difficult. A detailed history and examination is essential as soon as possible and a provisional diagnosis made based on the child's vital signs and clinical features.

Management of anaphylaxis

Once anaphylaxis is suspected, senior medical help should be summoned. The child should be reclined into a position of comfort (the supine position may help hypotension but could exacerbate breathing difficulties). The Resuscitation Council (UK) flowchart (Project Team of the Resuscitation Council (UK), 2001) (Fig. 9.1) summarizes the current recommendations for the management of anaphylaxis by first medical responders.

Oxygen

If available, oxygen should be administered at a rate of 10–15 litres per minute, preferably via a facemask with an oxygen reservoir bag. This will allow delivery of approximately 85% oxygen (Jevon, 2002).

Epinephrine (Adrenaline)

Epinephrine (adrenaline) is the most important drug in any severe anaphylactic reaction (Fisher, 1995). To be most effective it should be given promptly (Patel *et al.*, 1994). It reverses peripheral vasodilatation and reduces oedema (alpha receptor activity), dilates the airways, increases myocardial contractility and suppresses histamine and leukotriene release.

Using epinephrine (adrenaline) 1 : 1000 solution (100 μg/0.1 ml), the recommended dose is related to the child's age:

- >12 years: 500 μg i.m. (0.5 ml) (250 μg if the child is small or prepubertal)
- 6–12 years: 250 μg i.m. (0.25 ml)
- >6 months – 6 years: 120 μg i.m. (0.12 ml)
- <6 months: 50 μg i.m. (0.05 ml) – absolute accuracy of this small dose is not essential (Project Team of the Resuscitation Council (UK), 2001).

One dose of epinephrine (adrenaline) is usually sufficient (Wong *et al.*, 1999). However, it can be repeated after 5 minutes if there is no clinical improvement.

Sometimes several doses may be required (BNF, 2001).

The i.m. route is generally used for the administration of epinephrine (adrenaline) as it is relatively safe and adverse effects are rare. The more hazardous i.v. route is occasionally used, particularly if the child is in profound shock which is immediately life-threatening or in certain situations, e.g. anaesthesia. However, this route is only recommended for experienced

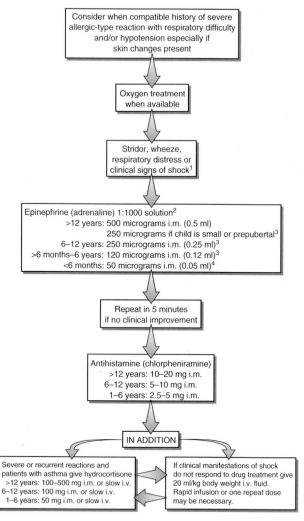

Consider when compatible history of severe allergic-type reaction with respiratory difficulty and/or hypotension especially if skin changes present

Oxygen treatment when available

Stridor, wheeze, respiratory distress or clinical signs of shock[1]

Epinephrine (adrenaline) 1:1000 solution[2]
>12 years: 500 micrograms i.m. (0.5 ml)
          250 micrograms if child is small or prepubertal[3]
6–12 years: 250 micrograms i.m. (0.25 ml)[3]
>6 months–6 years: 120 micrograms i.m. (0.12 ml)[3]
<6 months: 50 micrograms i.m. (0.05 ml)[4]

Repeat in 5 minutes if no clinical improvement

Antihistamine (chlorpheniramine)
>12 years: 10–20 mg i.m.
6–12 years: 5–10 mg i.m.
1–6 years: 2.5–5 mg i.m.

IN ADDITION

Severe or recurrent reactions and patients with asthma give hydrocortisone
>12 years: 100–500 mg i.m. or slow i.v.
6–12 years: 100 mg i.m. or slow i.v.
1–6 years: 50 mg i.m. or slow i.v.

If clinical manifestations of shock do not respond to drug treatment give 20 ml/kg body weight i.v. fluid. Rapid infusion or one repeat dose may be necessary.

Notes:
1. An inhaled beta$_2$-agonist such as salbutamol may be used as an adjunctive measure if bronchospasm is severe and does not respond rapidly to other treatment.
2. For profound shock judged immediately life threatening give CPR/ALS if necessary. Consider slow intravenous (i.v.) epinephrine (adrenaline) 1:10 000 solution. This is hazardous and is recommended only for an experienced practitioner who can also obtain i.v. access without delay. Note the different strength of epinephrine (adrenaline) is required for i.v. use.
3. For children who have been prescribed EpiPen, 150 micrograms can be given instead of 120 micrograms, and 300 micrograms can be given instead of 250 micrograms or 500 micrograms.
4. Absolute accuracy of the small dose is not essential.

Fig. 9.1 Project Team of the Resuscitation Council (UK) algorithm for the management of anaphylaxis in children by first medical responder (2001) (with permission of Aurum Pharmaceuticals).

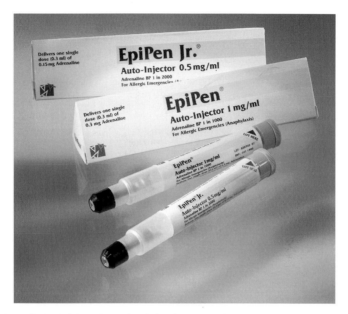

Fig. 9.2   Self-administration epinephrine (adrenaline).

practitioners who can secure i.v. access quickly. The 1 : 10 000 solution (100 μg/ml) of epinephrine (adrenaline) should be used in order to minimize complications following i.v. administration. Further dilution will increase its safety by reducing the risk of adverse effects (Brown, 1998). The ECG should be closely monitored.

If the child has been prescribed an EpiPen Jr. or EpiPen or similar (Fig. 9.2):

- EpiPen Jr. (150 μg) can be administered in children from 6 months to 6 years (instead of 120 μg)
- EpiPen (300 μg) can be administered in children >6 years (instead of 250 μg or 500 μg) (Project Team of the Resuscitation Council (UK), 2001).

(Additional fixed-dose self-administration syringes would facilitate more accurate dosing in young children (Simons *et al.*, 2002).)

Antihistamine

An antihistamine, e.g. chlorpheniramine (Piriton) should be used routinely in all anaphylactic reactions. Its use may be beneficial and is unlikely to be harmful (Project Team of the Resuscitation Council (UK), 1999). Care should be taken to avoid drug-induced hypotension. The recommended dose is related to the child's age:

- >12 years: 10–20 mg i.m.
- 6–12 years: 5–10 mg i.m.
- 1–6 years: 2.5–5 mg i.m.

Hydrocortisone

Hydrocortisone should be administered following severe anaphylactic reactions to help prevent late sequelae, particularly in asthmatics who have been on corticosteroid treatment previously. Again, care should be taken to avoid inducing further hypotension. The recommended dose is related to the child's age:

- >12 years: 100–500 mg i.m. or slow i.v.
- 6–12 years: 100 mg i.m. or slow i.v.
- 1–6 years: 50 mg i.m. or slow i.v.

Beta-agonist

An inhaled beta-agonist, e.g. salbutamol, may be used as an adjunctive measure if bronchospasm is severe and is not responding to standard treatment.

Fluids

If severe hypotension fails to respond rapidly to drug therapy, fluids (20 ml/kg) should be infused rapidly. A repeat rapid infusion may be required.

Cautions

- The possibility of misinterpreting a panic attack as anaphylaxis should be considered.
- Two strengths of epinephrine (adrenaline) are available; 1 : 1000 solution is used for i.m. injection, whereas the 1 : 10 000 solution is used for i.v. injection.
- The subcutaneous route for the administration of epinephrine (adrenaline) should not be utilized because absorption is considerably slower (Simons *et al.*, 1998).

Follow-up

Even if the reaction is only moderate, the child and parents should be warned of the possibility of an early recurrence of symptoms. Sometimes monitoring for 8–24 hours will be required, particularly when the reaction:

- is severe and is of slow onset because of idiopathic anaphylaxis
- occurs in a severe asthmatic
- is complicated by a severe asthmatic attack
- could be triggered again because further absorption of the allergen is possible.

Referring the child to an allergy clinic is essential. The cause of the anaphylaxis can be established by taking a structured allergy history and confirmed by the presence of specific IgE antibodies identified by skin-prick tests or a specific challenge to confirm or exclude the diagnosis (Clarke and Nasser, 2001).

Advice should be given concerning allergen avoidance. This is backed up by educating the parents or carers and relevant school personnel (Ewan and Clarke, 2001). Where appropriate, this should include the effective administration of epinephrine (adrenaline). The wearing of a Medic Alert bracelet may be required.

Summary

Anaphylaxis can be life threatening. This chapter has detailed the broad consensus guidelines by a Project Team of the Resuscitation Council (UK) (1999, 2001) on the appropriate emergency management of acute anaphylactic reactions by first medical responders. It is important to be able to recognize the clinical features of anaphylaxis and be familiar with the initial emergency management.

Chapter 10

Resuscitation in special situations

Introduction

Resuscitation in certain special situations, e.g. hypothermia, requires modification to the standard BLS and ALS guidelines in order to optimize the chances of survival.

These situations are often suspected by the history surrounding the event, knowledge of the common causes of cardiac arrest in the various age groups or prompt results from diagnostic investigations (American Heart Association, 2000).

The aim of this chapter is to understand the principles of resuscitation in special situations.

Objectives

At the end of the chapter the reader will be able to discuss the principles of cardiac management associated with the following special situations:

- hypothermia
- submersion
- acute severe asthma
- electrocution
- poisoning
- trauma.

Hypothermia

> **Hypothermia can mimic death and death can mimic hypothermia.**

Hypothermia can be defined as core body temperature <35°C. It can be classified as:

- mild (>32–<35°C)
- moderate (30–32°C)
- severe (<30°C) (Resuscitation Council (UK), 2000a).

Severe hypothermia is associated with a marked fall in cerebral blood flow and oxygen requirements, reduced cardiac output and decreased arterial pressure (Schneider, 1992). If there is rapid cooling prior to the development of hypoxaemia, decreased oxygen consumption and metabolism may precede the cardiac arrest and reduce organ ischaemia (Larach, 1995), exerting a protective effect on the brain and vital organs during cardiac arrest (Holzer *et al.*, 1997).

Core-temperature-related cardiac arrhythmias can complicate hypothermia: sinus bradycardia, atrial fibrillation, VF and then finally asystole (Resuscitation Council (UK), 2000a).

If the core temperature is < 30°C, defibrillation is unlikely to be effective until rewarming is accomplished (Southwick and Dalglish, 1980). In the presence of hypothermia, the heart may not respond to cardioactive drugs and pacemaker stimulation (Reuler, 1978). Metabolism of drugs is reduced; following repeated administration of drugs, concentrations can rise to toxic levels (Resuscitation Council (UK), 2000a).

Death should not be confirmed until the child's core temperature is at least 32°C or until efforts to raise the core temperature have failed (ALSG, 2001). Prolonged CPR may be required.

Resuscitation

All the principles of BLS and ALS apply to the hypothermic child (Resuscitation Council (UK), 2000a). However, some modifications to the approach are required:

- Palpate the pulse, look for signs of life and monitor ECG for up to 1 minute before diagnosing cardiac arrest – the vital signs may be difficult to detect (Schneider, 1992).
- Ventilate with warmed (40–46°C) and humidified oxygen – intubate the patient as soon as possible.
- Confirm hypothermia using a low-reading thermometer once CPR has been started.
- Prevent further heat loss if possible, e.g. remove wet clothing.
- In shock-refractory VF/VT (first three shocks are unsuccessful), defer further defibrillation attempts until core temperature > 30°C (Resuscitation Council (UK), 2000a).
- Cannulate a central or large proximal vein.
- Withhold drugs until core temperature > 30°C; then double the standard time intervals between drug administrations and use the lowest recommended drug doses. Only follow standard drug protocols once the core temperature returns towards normal (Resuscitation Council (UK), 2000a).
- Handle the child carefully – rough movement can precipitate cardiac arrhythmias (American Heart Association, 2000).

Rewarming

Although passive rewarming methods, e.g. warm blankets, warm environment, may suffice in cases of mild hypothermia (Kelly *et al.*, 2001), they will be ineffective if the patient is in cardiac arrest (Larach, 1995). In this situation active and rapid rewarming is essential (Carson, 1999).

Possible core temperature rewarming methods include:

- administration of warmed, humidified oxygen (42–46°C)

- infusion of warmed (43°C) normal saline centrally
- peritoneal lavage with warmed (43°C) potassium-free fluids (2 litres each lavage)
- extracorporeal blood-warming – preferred method because it ensures adequate support of oxygenation and ventilation while the core body temperature is gradually rewarmed (AHA and ILCOR, 2000).

The process of rewarming can cause vasodilatation and an expansion of vascular space. Large volumes of fluids may need to be administered. In addition, severe hyperkalaemia may also develop which will need correcting.

Submersion or near drowning

Death from drowning or near drowning is the third commonest cause of accidental death in the paediatric age group in the UK (after road traffic accidents and burns), often in private swimming pools, garden ponds and other inland waterways (ALSG, 2001).

Although survival following a prolonged submersion and a prolonged resuscitation attempt is rare, successful resuscitation associated with full neurological recovery is still possible in these circumstances (Siebke *et al.*, 1975; Southwick and Dalglish, 1980). If submersion occurs in icy water, the rapid development of hypothermia can provide some cerebral protection from hypoxia, particularly in small children (Quan *et al.*, 1992). Table 10.1 details the essential factors concerning a submersion incident.

The most significant and detrimental consequence of submersion is hypoxia, the duration of which is a critical factor in determining the

Table 10.1 Essential factors concerning the immersion incident (reproduced from Colquhoun *et al.* (1999) with kind permission of BMJ Books)

Length of time submerged	Favourable outcome associated with submersion for less than 5 minutes
Quality of immediate resuscitation	Favourable outcome if heart beat can be restored at once
Temperature of the water	Favourable outcome associated with immersion in ice-cold water (below 5°C), especially in infant victims
Shallow water	Consider fracture/dislocation of cervical spine
A buoyancy aid being used by the casualty	Likely to be profoundly hypothermic. Victim may not have aspirated water
Nature of the water (fresh or salt)	Ventilation–perfusion mismatch from fresh water inhalation more difficult to correct. Risk of infection from river water high. Consider leptospirosis

patient's outcome (AHA and ILCOR, 2000). Oxygenation, ventilation and perfusion are therefore of paramount importance.

Clearing the airways of aspirated water is not necessary (Rosen *et al.*, 1995). Approximately 10–15% of patients develop intense laryngeal spasm which protects the lungs from aspiration of water or gastric contents ('dry drowning') (Skinner and Vincent, 1997). Even if water is aspirated, it is only likely to be in small amounts and it is rapidly absorbed into the central circulation (Rosen *et al.*, 1995). Vomiting/regurgitation of gastric contents is common (Manolios and Mackie, 1988).

Responsiveness, either at the scene or on arrival at the A&E department, is a good prognostic indicator (Quan *et al.*, 1990). Poor prognostic indicators following submersion in children and adolescents include:

• submersion duration > 25 minutes
• resuscitation duration > 25 minutes
• pulseless cardiac arrest on arrival at the A&E department
• severe acidosis
• presence of VF/VT on the first recorded ECG (Quan and Kinder, 1992).

Resuscitation

All the principles of BLS and ALS apply when undertaking CPR on a child following submersion. However, some modifications to the approach are required:

• If cervical spine injury is suspected, apply jaw thrust, rather than head tilt/chin lift, to open the airway, and immobilize the child's spine using a cervical collar and spinal board or equivalent (cervical spine injury should be suspected if submersion was associated with a water sports or diving accident).
• Insert a nasogastric tube; empty and decompress the stomach – there is a risk of aspiration (ALSG, 2001).
• Administer antibiotics if there are signs of infection (more likely following submersion in a river).

In addition, the child may be hypothermic. The problems associated with undertaking CPR in the presence of hypothermia, together with specific modifications to the standard BLS and ALS protocols including rewarming, have already been discussed.

Acute severe asthma

Acute severe asthma attacks are normally reversible and related deaths should be considered avoidable (Resuscitation Council UK, 2000a). They are 10 times more common at night (Brenner *et al.*, 1999), and most asthma-related deaths occur outside hospital. National guidelines recommend aggressive treatment (oxygen, β_2-agonist, e.g. salbutamol, corticosteroids and aminophylline) of acute severe asthma to prevent deterioration to cardiac arrest.

Causes of cardiac arrest associated with acute severe asthma include:

• severe bronchospasm and mucous plugging (Molfino *et al.*, 1991)
• hypoxia-related cardiac arrhythmias
• tension pneumothorax.

Resuscitation

All the principles of BLS and ALS apply to undertaking CPR in a patient suffering a cardiac arrest following an acute severe asthma attack. However, some modifications to the approach are required:

• Intubate the trachea as soon as possible because high resistance in the airways can hinder ventilation; high ventilation pressures are usually required and gastric distension usually occurs during bag/valve/mask ventilation.
• Ensure prolonged inspiratory and expiratory times (8–10 inflations per minute) if necessary, in order to avoid high intrinsic positive end-expiratory pressure. A complication of this is sudden severe hypotension (AHA and ILCOR, 2000).
• Consider open chest cardiac massage (if expertise available) if chest compressions are ineffective because of a hyperinflated chest.

NB: **High airway pressures required for ventilation can cause a tension pneumothorax – clinical features include unilateral chest wall expansion, tracheal displacement to the opposite side and subcutaneous emphysema (AHA and ILCOR, 2000).**

Electrocution

Electrocution can result from domestic or industrial electricity, or from a lightning strike. Children account for 33% of all victims of electrocution (ALSG, 2001). Lightning strike injuries have a mortality rate of 30% with 70% of those who survive sustaining significant morbidity (Stewart, 2000).

Factors affecting severity of the injury

Factors that affect the severity of electrical injury include magnitude of energy delivered, voltage, resistance to current flow, type of current, duration of contact with the source of the current and current pathway (AHA and ILCOR, 2000).

Skin resistance, the most important factor impeding the flow of current, is reduced significantly by moisture, turning a minor injury into a life-threatening one (Wallace, 1991).

There are two types of current:

• *Direct current (DC)* – present in batteries and lightning; the current flows in one direction for the duration of discharge. It induces one strong muscular contraction that often throws the casualty away from the current source (Fontanarosa, 1993).

- *Alternating current (AC)* – present in most household and commercial sources of electricity. Contact with it may cause tetanic skeletal muscle contractions, preventing self-release from the current source (AHA and ILCOR, 2000). The repetitive frequency of AC increases the risk of current flow through the myocardium during the vulnerable refractory period of the cardiac cycle, which can cause VF (Geddes *et al.*, 1986).

Transthoracic current flow (hand-to-hand current pathway) is more likely to be fatal than a vertical current pathway (hand-to-foot) or a straddle current pathway (foot-to-foot) (Thompson and Ashwal, 1983).

Clinical effects on the child

Electrocution injuries result from the direct effects of the current on cell membranes and vascular smooth muscle, and the production of heat energy as it passes through body tissues (AHA and ILCOR, 2000).

Cardiac arrest, VF or asystole, is the primary cause of death following electrocution (Homma *et al.*, 1990). Respiratory arrest can be caused by a variety of different mechanisms:

- passage of electric current through the brain inhibiting the respiratory centre in the medulla
- tetanic contraction of the diaphragm and chest wall during exposure to the current
- prolonged paralysis of the respiratory muscles (AHA and ILCOR, 2000).

Electrical injuries often cause related trauma, e.g. cervical spine injury (Epperly and Stewart, 1989) and skin burns.

Resuscitation

All the principles of BLS and ALS apply to undertaking CPR in a patient suffering a cardiac arrest following electrocution. However, some modifications to the approach are required:

- If applicable ensure that the environment is safe and there is no electrocution risk to the team.
- Immobilize the cervical spine and apply jaw thrust, rather than head tilt/chin lift to open the airway.
- Intubate early, particularly if there are burns to the face, mouth or neck (soft-tissue oedema may rapidly develop and obstruct the airway) (Resuscitation Council (UK), 2000a).
- Monitor breathing and provide assisted ventilation as required (muscular paralysis may persist for up to 30 minutes following electrocution) (Resuscitation Council (UK), 2000a).
- Remove any smouldering clothes or shoes to prevent further thermal injury.
- Administer sufficient fluids to maintain adequate diuresis to excrete by-products of tissue destruction including potassium and myoglobin (Cooper, 1995).

- Continue resuscitation for prolonged periods if required.
- Request surgical expertise if there are severe thermal injuries.

Poisoning

Fortunately death from poisoning in the paediatric age group is declining, particularly following the introduction of child-resistant drug containers in the 1970s (although 20% of children < 5 years can open them) (ALSG, 2001). However, suspected poisoning still accounts for approximately 40 000 attendances in A&E departments in England and Wales each year (ALSG, 2001).

With some poisoning agents, cardiac arrest results from direct cardiotoxicity while with others it is secondary to respiratory arrest caused by CNS depression or aspiration of gastric contents (Nelson and Hoffman, 1996). Pulseless electrical activity (PEA), a common complication of ingestion of drugs with negative inotropic properties, carries a far better prognosis than when associated with a primary cardiac cause (Resuscitation Council (UK), 2000a).

Resuscitation

All the principles of BLS and ALS apply to undertaking CPR in a patient suffering a cardiac arrest following poisoning. However, some modifications to the approach are required:

- If necessary, ensure relevant precautions are taken if poisoning is due to gas, corrosives, etc.
- Intubate the child as soon as possible, as there is a high incidence of pulmonary aspiration of gastric contents associated with poisoning.
- If possible, identify the poison(s) ingested: information from the child's relatives, friends and ambulance crew may be of help. Also examine the child for needle puncture marks, tablet bottles/sachets, odours, corrosion around the mouth.
- Access TOXBASE or telephone the National Poisons Information Service if specialist help and advice are required – follow local protocols.
- Reverse the effects of the toxin if possible by administering the appropriate antidote.
- Provide intensive supportive therapy, correcting hypoxia, acid–base and electrolyte imbalances.
- Continue resuscitation for prolonged periods if required, as the poison may be metabolized or excreted during this time (Resuscitation Council (UK), 2000a).

Specific poisons and antidotes

Opiates (including methadone)

Clinical features include respiratory depression, pinpoint pupils and unconsciousness. Naloxone remains the treatment of choice to reverse narcotic toxicity (American Academy of Pediatrics Committee on Drugs,

1990). The recommended dose is 0.1 mg/kg i.v. (maximum 2 mg in one dose) (American Academy of Pediatrics Committee, 1989). Care should be taken to ensure adequate ventilation prior to administration of naloxone because ventricular arrhythmias may occur in the presence of hypercapnia (Osterwalder, 1996). As the action of naloxone lasts for approximately 45–70 minutes compared to several hours for opiates (AHA and ILCOR, 2000), repeated doses may be required.

Tricyclic antidepressants

These can lead to convulsions and cardiac arrhythmias. Tricyclic anti-depressant toxicity can result in pre-terminal sinus bradycardia and AV block with junctional or ventricular broad-complex escape beats (Ettinger *et al.*, 1974). A QRS complex > 0.16 s (four small squares) is considered a predictor of serious toxicity (ALSG, 2001). Most life-threatening complications occur within 6 hours of ingestion (Resuscitation Council (UK), 2000a).

Alkalization (pH – at least 7.45, ideally 7.50) is recommended because it will reduce the toxic effects on the heart (ALSG, 2001). It can be achieved by hyperventilation and the administration of sodium bicarbonate (1–2 mmol/kg i.v.) (ALSG, 2001). Sodium bicarbonate can also help to suppress cardiac arrhythmias and reverse hypotension (Hoffman *et al.*, 1993; McCabe *et al.*, 1998).

If cardiac arrhythmias do not respond to the sodium bicarbonate, an anti-arrhythmic drug may be required. However, guidance from a poisons unit is advisable (ALSG, 2001) because some are contraindicated in this situation, e.g. amiodarone (Shanon and Liebelt, 1998). Lidocaine (lignocaine) is often considered (American Heart Association, 2000), though its use is controversial (Derlet *et al.*, 1991).

Convulsions should be treated, initially with lorazepam 0.1 mg/kg i.v. (rectal diazepam if unable to secure i.v. access) (ALSG, 2001). Hypotension should be treated with volume expansion and with an inotrope if necessary, e.g. noradrenaline (norepinephrine) (ALSG, 2001).

Trauma

Poor resuscitation technique is a major cause of preventable death associated with paediatric trauma (McKoy and Bell, 1983). Common contributing factors include failure to:

- open and maintain a clear airway
- provide appropriate fluid resuscitation in a head injury
- recognize and treat internal haemorrhage (Dykes *et al.*, 1989).

Causes of cardiac arrest in a child with trauma include hypoxia, tension pneumothorax, hypovolaemia and cardiac tamponade.

Resuscitation

All the principles of BLS and ALS apply to undertaking CPR in a patient suffering a cardiac arrest following trauma. However, some modifications

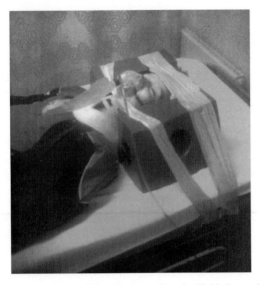

Fig. 10.1   Cervical spine immobilization (reproduced with kind permission from the Advanced Life Support Group, Manchester, UK).

to the approach are required:

- Perform jaw thrust not head tilt/chin lift to open the airway.
- Immobilize the cervical spine (Fig. 10.1) – difficult in young children when trying to maintain the head in the neutral position (Curran *et al.*, 1995). Cervical spine injury is less common in children than in adults (Kewalramani *et al.*, 1980). It is more commonly associated with road traffic accidents and falls from a height (Ruge *et al.*, 1988).
- Exclude tension pneumothorax when ventilating.
- Site two wide-bore cannulae and administer volume replacement if indicated – a transfusion of 10–15 ml/kg of blood may be required (American Heart Association, 2000).
- Request surgical expertise and treat any life-threatening problems.
- Suspect thoracic injury (often no external evidence) if there is a history of thoracoabdominal trauma or if ventilation is difficult (American Heart Association, 2000).

Summary

Resuscitation in certain special situations requires modification of the standard BLS and ALS guidelines if the chances of survival are to be.optimized. The key principles of resuscitation in these special situations have been discussed.

Chapter 11

Post-resuscitation care

Introduction

Many children who survive cardiac arrest unfortunately die hours or days later from multiple organ failure (ALSG, 2001). The aim of post-resuscitation care is to achieve and maintain homeostasis, which will maximize the possibility of recovery (ALSG, 2001).

However, post-resuscitation care is complex, requiring knowledge and expertise in the evaluation of all organ systems, assessment and monitoring of physiological functions and management of multi-organ failure (American Heart Association, 2000). In addition, transfer to definitive care will be required.

The aim of this chapter is to understand the principles of post-resuscitation care.

Objectives

At the end of the chapter the reader will be able to:

- list the goals of post-resuscitation care
- outline the initial assessment priorities
- describe measures to limit secondary cerebral damage
- outline the guidelines for referral to a paediatric intensive care unit
- discuss the standards for the retrieval of critically ill children
- list the basic principles of safe transport.

Goals of post-resuscitation care

The goals of post-resuscitation care are to:

- perform an initial assessment of the child's vital signs and prevent a further cardiac arrest
- preserve cerebral function
- limit damage to vital organs
- identify and treat the cause of illness
- transfer the patient to definitive care in the best physiological state.

Initial assessment and treatment priorities

The initial management priorities involve opening and maintaining a clear airway, ensuring adequate ventilation and ensuring adequate circulation.

Airway

The child's airway may be at risk due to reduced conscious level or depressed gag reflex. Prompt assessment of the child's airway should therefore be undertaken: check the mouth (signs and treatment of a partially or completely obstructed airway have been discussed in detail in Ch. 5) and apply suction using a rigid wide-bore cannula (Yankauer) if required. Check the child's level of consciousness. A tracheal tube may need to be inserted to secure the airway and facilitate mechanical ventilation. Correct tracheal tube placement, together with tube patency, should be verified and regularly monitored. If the clinical state of an intubated child deteriorates, remember the mnemonic *DOPE* (see p. 62).

Breathing

Inadequate ventilation leading to prolonged hypoxia will increase the risk of a further cardiac arrest and could contribute to further neurological damage. The child's breathing should therefore be accurately assessed and supported if necessary. Methods of assessing breathing and ventilation include:

- Look, listen and feel for signs of breathing.
- Examine the child's chest. Look for symmetrical and bilateral chest movement. Auscultate the chest to assess bilateral air entry.
- Pulse oximetry, though the readings can be unreliable if there is poor skin perfusion or if the child is hypothermic (Jevon and Ewens, 2002).
- Arterial blood gas analysis (and acid–base) (Fig. 11.1).
- Capnography – helps to avoid hypoventilation and hyperventilation (Tobias *et al.*, 1996).
- Chest X-ray.

If the child is breathing adequately, high concentrations of oxygen should be administered via a non-rebreathe mask (Fig. 11.2). If the child is not breathing, mechanical ventilation should continue using available equipment, e.g. bag/valve/mask device, portable ventilator. If a mechanical ventilator is being used, the recommended initial tidal volumes are 7–10 ml/kg, sufficient to achieve visible chest rise and audible breath sounds over the distal lung fields (American Heart Association, 2000). The aim is to ensure that oxygen saturation is maintained at >95% (ALSG, 2001).

A nasogastric tube may need to be inserted to decompress the stomach (gastric inflation often associated with bag/valve/mask ventilation can cause diaphragmatic splinting) and allow aspiration of gastric contents.

Circulation

Circulatory dysfunction frequently occurs following resuscitation from cardiac arrest (Lucking *et al.*, 1986; ALSG, 2001). Common causes include:

- myocardial depression due to hypoxia, acidosis and toxins
- hypovolaemia

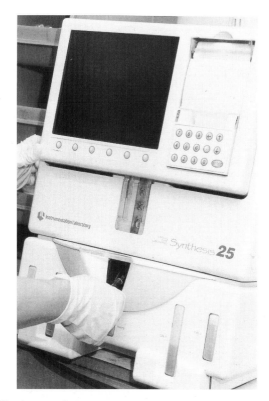

Fig. 11.1 Blood gas analyser.

- acid–base disturbance
- electrolyte abnormality
- loss of peripheral vascular tone.

The maintenance of adequate cardiac output and oxygen delivery to the tissues is paramount if multi-organ function is to be preserved (American Heart Association, 2000). Clinical assessment of circulation and cardiac output should therefore be carried out.

Clinical signs of inadequate cardiac output and poor tissue perfusion (discussed in more detail in Ch. 3) include:

- tachycardia
- delayed capillary refill (>2 seconds)
- cool and pale peripheries
- weak or absent distal pulses
- decreased urine output
- altered neurological status (e.g. confusion, agitation and decrease in conscious level)
- hypotension (late sign).

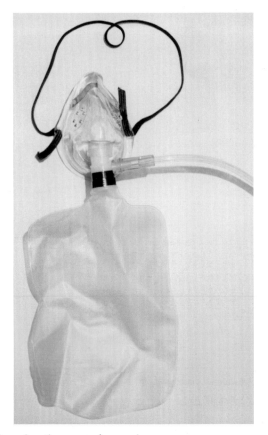

Fig. 11.2 Non-rebreathe oxygen facemask.

NB: **Blood pressure may be normal despite the presence of shock (American Heart Association, 2000).**

The pulse should be noted and ECG monitoring started. Blood pressure measurements should be recorded, together with adequacy of peripheral perfusion (temperature, colour and capillary refill of the peripheries). The neurological status and urine output should also be closely monitored.

The insertion of an arterial cannula will allow continuous arterial blood pressure measurements and repeated sampling for arterial blood gas analysis. Central venous pressure monitoring may be required and urine output should be closely monitored. A pulmonary artery catheter may sometimes be inserted to monitor pulmonary capillary wedge pressure and cardiac output (Ceneviva *et al.*, 1998), though non-invasive Doppler techniques may be a better alternative. Fluids and inotropes (e.g. dobutamine, dopamine or adrenaline (epinephrine)) may be required, depending on haemodynamic measurements. Expert advice should be sought.

Neurological assessment

A baseline neurological assessment should be undertaken and documented using the Glasgow Coma Score (GCS) or Paediatric GCS (<4 years) (Fig. 11.3). The GCS, originally developed to grade the severity and outcome in traumatic head injury (Teasdale and Jennett, 1974), is now used as an unvalidated tool for the description of states of consciousness from all pathologies (ALSG, 2001).

The GCS will provide a benchmark for further assessments. However, in the post-resuscitation phase, pupil size can be affected by CO_2 retention, atropine, adrenaline (epinephrine) and local ischaemia to the front of the eye (Oakley and Redmond, 1999).

Investigations

If possible, it is important to ascertain the cause of the cardiopulmonary arrest so that any appropriate treatment can then be started. The child's history and events leading up to the cardiopulmonary arrest may be significant. A number of investigations will need to be carried out (Box 11.1).

Renal function

Renal perfusion should be maximized and renal tubular patency maintained (by: ensuring adequate urine flow) by:

- maintaining adequate oxygenation
- maintaining adequate cardiac output
- administering (judiciously) diuretics to maintain urine output >1 ml/ kg/hour
- correcting any electrolyte and acid–base imbalances (ALSG, 2001).

Metabolic function

Infants and children have high glucose requirements (particularly when seriously ill) and low glycogen stores. As hypoglycaemia is frequently observed in the post-resuscitation period, blood glucose levels should therefore be checked and closely monitored (Fig. 11.4).

Box 11.1   Post-resuscitation investigations (not exhaustive)

- Arterial blood gas analysis
- Chest X-ray
- Full blood count
- Biochemistry (urea, electrolytes, glucose)

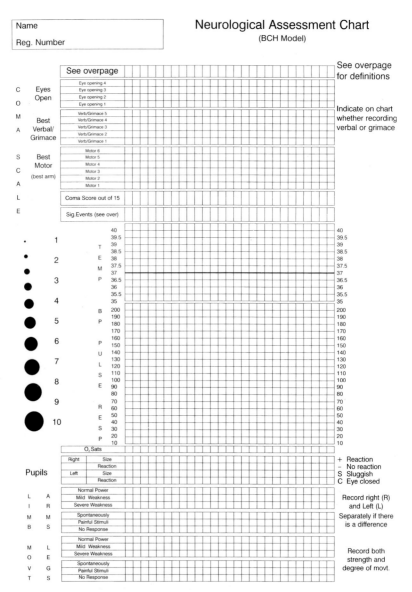

Fig. 11.3a Modified Paediatric Coma Scale (reproduced with kind permission of Birmingham Children's Hospital) (*cont'd on p.125*).

Modified Paediatric Coma Scale
Adapted by Tatman, Warren, Powell, Whitehouse & Noons '97
Birmingham Children's Hospital NHS Trust

Painful stimuli should be created by applying pressure on the side of the finger sufficient to evoke a response (avoid pressing on the nail bed).*

In specific circumstances it may be necessary to apply central stimuli (ie supraorbital pressure).

Always score the best response (e.g. if unclear, or if there is a difference between right and left sides).

Score NA (not applicable) when there is for example brainstem, cervical spine cord or neuromuscular junction (neuromuscular block) impairment. Score C for eyes closed by swelling or bandage.

Use Grimace score if there is no verbal (audible), response i.e. if Silent (S) or intubated (T).

*Frawley P. (1990) Neurological Observations NT 86 (35) pp 29-34

Adult/Child according to usual ability

Eye opening (E)
E4. Spontaneous
E3. To verbal stimuli
E2. To painful stimuli
E1. None to painful stimuli
C. Eyes closed by swelling/bandage

Verbal (V)
V5. Orientated (person, place or address)
V4. Confused
V3. Inappropriate words
V2. Inappropriate sounds
V1. None
S. Silent or mute
T. Intubated

Grimace (see above for usage)
G5. Spontaneous normal facial/oro-motor activity,
G4. Less than usual spontaneous ability or only response to touch stimuli.
G3. Vigorous grimace to pain.
G2. Mild grimace to pain.
G1. No response to pain.
NA. Not applicable.

Motor (M)
M6. Obeys commands
M5. Localise to painful stimuli
M4. Withdraws to painful stimuli
M3. Abnormal flexion to pain (de corticate)
M2. Abnormal extension to pain (de cerebrate)
M1. No response to pain
NA. Not applicable.

Child/Infant

As for older child

V.5 Alert, babbles, coos, words or sentences to normal ability.
V.4 Less than usual ability or spontaneous irritable cry.
V.3 Cries inappropriately
V.2 Occasionally whimpers and/or moans
V1.as for older child
"
"

As for older children

M6. Or normal spontaneous movements
M5. Or withdraws to touch
M4. As for older children
"
"
"
"

Fig. 11.3b Modified Paediatric Coma Scale (*cont'd*).

Hypoglycaemia should be treated with 0.5 g/kg dextrose (5 ml/kg of 10% dextrose) (ALSG, 2001), ideally with a continuous infusion rather than bolus therapy, which will hopefully avoid hyperglycaemia and its associated detrimental effects (American Heart Association, 2000).

Hyperglycaemia should be avoided as it will increase cerebral metabolism (Oakley and Redmond, 1999) and may have detrimental effects on neurological outcome (Pulsineli *et al.*, 1982; Sieber and Traystman, 1992; Cherian *et al.*, 1997). In addition, hyperglycaemia will cause a sharp rise in serum osmolality, which may result in osmotic diuresis (American Heart Association, 2000).

Metabolic acidosis usually develops during a cardiac arrest, resulting in a low pH (acidaemia), low bicarbonate and a base deficit; the normal physiological response is an increase in minute ventilation (respiratory compensation) (Resuscitation Council (UK), 2000a). Certainly, blood gas and acid–base abnormalities should be controlled initially by adequate ventilation and restoration of renal function (Oakley and Redmond, 1999).

The role of sodium bicarbonate in the post-resuscitation period in children with documented acidosis is not clear (American Heart Association, 2000). The routine use of sodium bicarbonate to treat acidosis is no longer recommended, except in certain situations, e.g. tricyclic overdose (Hoffman *et al.*, 1993), hyperkalaemia (Ettinger *et al.*, 1974).

If administered, the recommended dose is 1 mmol/kg (1 ml/kg of 8.4% solution) (ALSG, 2001). Adequate ventilation must be maintained to avoid respiratory acidosis (the bicarbonate ion is excreted as carbon dioxide via the lungs). The blood pH and base excess should also be monitored, though the accuracy of arterial blood gas analysis during cardiac arrest or severe shock has been questioned (Weil *et al.*, 1986; Steedman and Robertson, 1992).

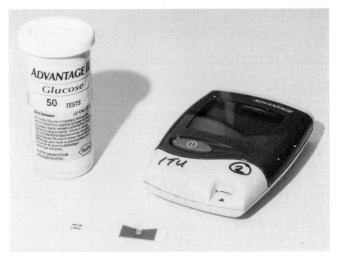

Fig. 11.4   Blood glucose monitoring: testing strips and testing meter.

Temperature control

Temperature normalization is important because both hyperthermia and hypothermia may be harmful:

Hyperthermia   This increases the cerebral metabolic rate (8% for every 1°C rise in temperature), potentially creating an imbalance between oxygen demand and oxygen supply (European Resuscitation Council, 1998). This may impair cerebral recovery.

Hypothermia   Although induced hypothermia is used effectively during certain surgical procedures, e.g. cardiac surgery, there is as yet no evidence that it is beneficial in the post-resuscitation period. Cardiac arrhythmias, a fall in cardiac output and increased susceptibility to infection are recognized detrimental effects of hypothermia (European Resuscitation Council, 1998).

The following is therefore recommended in respect of temperature normalization (ALSG, 2001):

- Monitor the child's temperature (Fig. 11.5).
- No routine use of hypothermia in the post-resuscitation situation.
- If the child's core temperature < 33°C, rewarm to 34°C.
- Treat hyperthermia with active cooling.
- Control shivering (it increases metabolic demand), e.g. with sedation or neuromuscular blockade.

Measures to minimize secondary cerebral damage

One of the aims of post-resuscitation care is to prevent further (secondary) cerebral damage. This can be achieved by maintaining cerebral blood flow,

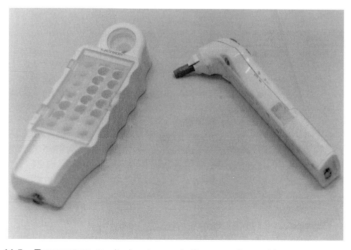

Fig. 11.5   Temperature monitoring: tympanic thermometer and lens covers.

achieving normal cellular homeostasis and reducing cerebral metabolic needs (ALSG, 2001). The Advanced Life Support Group (ALSG, 2001) has identified the following practical measures to minimize secondary cerebral damage:

- Maintain adequate oxygenation.
- Maintain adequate circulation, using inotropes and fluids as necessary.
- Correct any electrolyte imbalances.
- Correct any acid–base disturbance.
- Normalize the blood sugar.
- Normalize body temperature.
- Administer adequate analgesia and sedation.
- Control convulsions.
- Reduce intracranial pressure.

Guidelines for referral to a paediatric intensive care unit

The Paediatric Intensive Care Society (PICS) in its 'Standards Document 2001' has issued guidelines for referral to a paediatric intensive care unit (PICU) (Fig. 11.6). All purchasers and providers of healthcare and allied services should be aware of the guidelines for PICU referral. In addition, duty managers and consultants in all hospitals should be aware of how to contact the lead centre for paediatric intensive care. The guidelines are as follows:

- Intensive care admission must involve consultant-to-consultant referral between the consultant responsible for the patient's care in the referring centre and the consultant in charge of the PICU.
- The duty consultant in charge of the PICU at the lead centre must be available for consultation at all times.
- Consultation between referring unit and lead centre must remain possible irrespective of the availability of an intensive care bed at the lead centre.
- The management of patients discussed with the lead centre remains the responsibility of the referring team until care is taken over by a retrieval team or, in other circumstances, after the patient has been transferred.
- Institutions without intensive care facilities on site should, by default, make all their paediatric intensive care referrals to a lead centre.
- Institutions with a paediatric or general intensive care unit that are not lead centres for paediatric intensive care should refer patients to the lead centre if intensive care is likely to be required for more than 24 hours or if it is indicated because of failure or a need for support involving more than one organ system.
- PICS regards the 'procedures' listed in Box 11.2 as being 'intensive care dependent'. Under normal circumstances, when required they should usually be performed on children within a paediatric critical care environment.

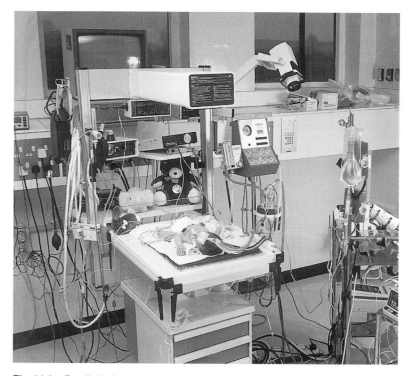

Fig. 11.6 Paediatric intensive care unit.

Box 11.2 Intensive care dependent procedures (from PICs, 2001, with permission)

- Nasopharyngeal and endotracheal intubation
- Endotracheal continuous positive airway pressure (endotracheal CPAP) (acute, short and medium term)
- Artificial/mechanical ventilation (acute, short and medium term)
- Continuous invasive cardiovascular monitoring (e.g. central venous or arterial line or Swan–Ganz catheter)
- Use of antiarrhythmic, inotropic or vasoactive drug infusions
- Acute renal support (haemodialysis, haemofiltration, plasmafiltration and peritoneal dialysis)
- Cardioversion or DC countershock
- Acute or external cardiac pacing
- Mechanical circulatory support
- Intracranial pressure monitoring
- Complex intravenous nutrition and drug scheduling
- Complex anticonvulsant therapy
- Frequent or pressurized infusions of blood products
- Active or forced diuresis
- Induced hypothermia
- Balloon tamponade of oesophageal varices
- Emergency thoraco- or pericardiocentesis

Box 11.3   Indications for PICU admission (Paediatric Intensive Care Society, 2001)

- Advanced respiratory support (i.e. acute, short-, or medium-term mechanical ventilation) required
- Intensive care dependent procedure (Box 11.2) required
- Symptoms or evidence of shock, respiratory distress or respiratory depression present
- Potential to develop airway compromise
- Unexplained deterioration in level of consciousness
- Resuscitation has been required or is on-going
- Significant injury
- After prolonged surgery or any surgical procedure that is medium or high risk or of a specialist nature, even if this surgery is elective
- Potential for or actual severe metabolic derangement, fluid or electrolyte imbalance
- Acute organ (or organ-system) failure
- Established chronic disease (or organ-system failure) with severe acute clinical deterioration or secondary failure in another organ system
- One-to-one nursing required because of the severity of an acute or chronic illness

---

- Indications for paediatric intensive care admission are listed in Box 11.3.
- Any decision to refer a patient outside the normal referral region for paediatric intensive care should involve consultation between the referring consultant and the consultant in charge of the lead centre.

Standards for retrieval of critically ill children

The PICS in its Standards Document 2001 has made recommendations in respect of standards for the retrieval of critically ill children:

Applicability

- Lead centres should be funded for a retrieval service (24 hours a day, 7 days a week) for children who require intensive care within the agreed catchment area whenever they have an available bed.
- Supra-regional transfer services should be separately funded as part of the funding of the supra-regional service, as distinct from regional lead centre activity.
- In the presence of a separate, centralized designated paediatric intensive care retrieval service, the lead centre should ensure/endorse the standard and training of the staff providing the service.
- Centres providing supra-regional services should have protocols in place for the transfer of such children from their referral centres.
- Primary transport (by referring hospitals) will be necessary for some conditions such as expanding intracranial haematoma and severe thoracic vascular trauma.
- Standards for primary transport (by referring hospitals) should be agreed with the lead centre or specialist unit and the circumstances in which they should be used should be clearly defined.

Availability

- Under normal circumstances lead centres are obligated to retrieve patients referred and accepted for intensive care on their units. They are not obligated to transfer them elsewhere in the event of supra-regional referral or lack of available beds.
- The local lead centre retrieval service should be available on at least 95% of days with a back-up plan for those occasions when the service is not available.
- In the presence of a separate, centralized designated paediatric intensive care retrieval service, this team should undertake the transfer of patients outside the normally served geographic region if required to do so for reasons of supra-regional referral or lack of available beds.
- There should be equity of access to the retrieval service.

Medical staffing

- The retrieval service is staffed as a remote intensive care bed requiring 1:1 nursing and its own medical staff member.
- The service should be consultant led and where necessary consultant provided.
- During a retrieval performed by a paediatric intensive care consultant, the PICU should be covered by another paediatric intensive care consultant.
- The lead centre paediatric intensive care consultants are responsible for deciding which medical staff are appropriately trained and experienced to carry out retrieval and to agree the rota as appropriate.
- Training in paediatric intensive care transport must include supervised transports (i.e. accompanied by the trainer).
- The decision as to what level of medical staff to despatch for retrieval should be made in consultation with the referring consultant and assessed as part of the referral for intensive care.
- Under normal circumstances if a primary transport is required (i.e. by staff from the referral hospital) then the medical staff member involved must be appropriately trained with general intensive care and paediatric airway expertise.

Nurse staffing

- The establishment for nursing at the lead centre should allow for a transport trained nurse to be available to undertake retrieval duties 24 hours a day. They will therefore not be included in this baseline establishment.
- The lead nurse at the lead centre is responsible for deciding which nurses are appropriately trained and experienced to carry out retrieval and to agree the rota as appropriate. These are expected to be ENB 415 (or equivalent) trained.
- Training in paediatric intensive care transport must include supervised transports (i.e. accompanied by the trainer).

- If a primary transport is required (i.e. by staff from the referral hospital) then the accompanying staff member involved must be a senior/experienced intensive care or A&E nurse or operating department assistant.

Environment and support services

- Parents/carers should be given as much information about the retrieval service as early as possible in the referring centre.
- Parents/carers/guardians should be told that it is unlikely they will be able to accompany the child during transfer.
- Referring hospitals are obligated to provide transport to the lead centre for parents of critically ill children being transferred.
- Advice about travel arrangements to the lead centre should be available for other family members.
- Wherever possible, the child should undergo one retrieval journey only.

Equipment and facilities

- The retrieval team should be able to retrieve the child from a designated critical care area within the referring hospital, which should be agreed with the lead centre.
- The retrieval team should be fully equipped and able to deal with children of all ages.
- Retrieval teams should not need to rely upon paramedic ambulance services.

Quality and management of services

- Compatible protocols should be developed between the lead centre and referring hospitals.
- Arrangements for contacting the retrieval team should be clearly displayed within critical care areas at referring hospitals.
- The lead centre must provide adequate information to referring hospitals.
- The referring hospitals must undertake to provide full clinical information to the intended receiving team.
- The retrieval service should be continuously audited and data collected on all referrals and retrievals. This includes referrals that do not result in transfer, and records should include the nature of any medical or nursing advice given by the lead centre.
- Critical incident recording should be included in retrieval records and audit.

Operational issues

- Primary transport for emergencies such as neurosurgical intervention for an expanding intracranial haematoma, should not be deferred or re-routed as a result of actual, declared or suspected availability of a paediatric intensive care bed. The patient should be immediately transferred to the nearest centre capable of performing the life-saving procedure and a paediatric intensive care bed should then be sought when the patient's condition has been stabilized, e.g. postoperatively.

- By its very nature, retrieval exposes the staff (and patient) to additional personal and professional hazards. The service must be appropriately insured and indemnified with written confirmation of such, before retrieval is offered. Furthermore the establishment of a paediatric intensive care retrieval service has considerable implications for ambulance and other emergency services which must be consulted during the planning and preparation phases of establishing a service. The likely modes of transport should be determined in advance and their sources and availability identified and negotiated. Depending upon local circumstances and the nature of the individual case, the choice of vehicle may be different for outward and return journeys.

- Under normal circumstances, paediatric intensive care retrieval is a 'secondary transfer' occurring with less desperate urgency than in a primary transfer after the patient has been resuscitated and stabilized. The retrieval service cannot provide timely assistance with the initial resuscitation. The onus of responsibility remains with the referring hospital to initiate and continue competent resuscitation and stabilization from the outset until handing over to the retrieval team.

- The referral of a patient to a PICU must be on the basis of a referring consultant talking directly to the duty paediatric intensive care consultant.

- There should be a dedicated phone line on the PICU for arranging retrievals, the telephone number of which should be distributed to hospitals in the catchment area. Details of the patient's age, history, (likely) diagnosis, vital signs and precise location should be documented along with a record of any advice given and contact telephone numbers.

- Transport/retrieval staff must be skilled paediatric intensive care practitioners who have received specific additional training in transport as well as in intensive care.

- The transport team should not be dependent upon paramedic support from the ambulance service.

- A clear hierarchy is necessary amongst the retrieval team with a single team leader. This individual is in charge of the patient, not the transport vehicle. Upon their arrival at the referring centre and after a concise but comprehensive medical and nursing handover, the team take over clinical management and assume responsibility for the patient who is then prepared for transport. The patient must not be moved until the retrieval team leader is satisfied that preparation for transport has been adequate.

Basic principles of safe transport

Meticulous attention to the initial assessment and resuscitation of the child, together with the appropriate emergency management, will reduce the risk of transport-related morbidity and mortality (ALSG, 2001). Basic principles of safe transport apply to the movement of all sick children, whether within or between hospitals and whether or not a specialist retrieval team are involved; they include:

- stabilizing the child prior to transport (Henning, 1992)
- securing the airway, ensuring adequate ventilation and adequate circulation
- correcting any hypoglycaemia
- securing i.v. lines etc.
- communicating effectively with receiving hospital or department
- communicating effectively with other members of the team
- ensuring adequate transport is arranged
- organizing appropriately trained staff to escort
- ensuring appropriate emergency and monitoring equipment is assembled – all in working order, batteries fully charged, full oxygen cylinders, etc.
- monitoring airway, breathing and circulation and maintaining temperature (preventing hypothermia)
- ensuring appropriate documentation is taken
- ensuring adequate communication with parents.

Summary

Post-resuscitation care initially involves maintaining a clear airway, ensuring adequate ventilation and oxygenation with 100% oxygen and ensuring adequate circulation. In addition, measures should be taken to minimize secondary cerebral damage. Guidelines for referral to a paediatric intensive care unit and the standards for the retrieval of critically ill children have been discussed.

Chapter 12

Bereavement

Introduction

For any healthcare professional, dealing with the death of a child is a very emotive situation. When a failed resuscitation, the unknown cause of death and deeply traumatized relatives are added to the scenario, a child's death can be a deeply distressing and stressful event for staff to deal with.

The successful management of such a tragic and distressing situation requires good team work, effective communication between all those involved, set protocols to follow and support of staff. It is essential that family-centred care remains the focus and priority of those delivering the care.

The aim of this chapter is to understand the general principles of managing bereavement. If a more comprehensive and detailed account is required, this can be found elsewhere (Wright, 1996).

Objectives

At the end of this chapter the reader will be able to:

- describe an ideal layout for the family room
- discuss the principles of breaking bad news
- discuss the principles of telephone notification of family members
- outline the practical arrangements following a death
- discuss the importance of written guidelines and policies
- discuss the issues involved with family members witnessing resuscitation.

Ideal layout for the family room

The family room should be spacious, well lit and if possible have a window to the outside. This will help to reduce parents/relatives' concerns about being claustrophobic and isolated (Bury Medical Audit, 1994). In addition, the room should ideally have the following:

- comfortable domestic chairs and sofas, including provision for people with special needs
- ashtrays
- telephone with direct dial-in and dial-out facilities and telephone directories
- wash basin with soap, towel, mirror, freshen-up pack and tissues
- television/radio available but not prominent

- hot and cold drinks, refrigerator, kettle and a non-institutional tea/coffee set
- books and toys for children
- access to toilet facilities (British Association of A&E Medicine and the Royal College of Nursing, 1994).

Breaking bad news

Allocation of an experienced nurse

The allocation of an experienced nurse to care for family members is recommended. This nurse should:

- be familiar with resuscitation procedures and terminology
- have good communication skills
- have good counselling skills
- be able to undertake this role unsupervised (Rattrie, 2000).

Who should tell the relatives

If the family are not present when the child dies, or if they arrive after the death, someone will have to break the news to them. This should be done at the earliest opportunity, thus saving them from waiting in vain and hoping for good news. It is essential that the person breaking the bad news (usually a doctor) knows the child's name and has been present at the resuscitation; he or she should be accompanied by the nurse who has been caring for the family.

Preparation

Adequate preparation is essential. All the information relevant to the child, including medical and resuscitation details, should be gathered together. Self-preparation, e.g. washing hands, checking clothing for blood, is also important. The names of the closest family members should be sought.

Good communication techniques

Good communication techniques include:

- introducing yourself and colleague(s)
- confirming they are members of the correct family and identifying who are the closest members (usually the parents)
- sitting down in order to be at the same level as the relatives
- establishing and maintaining eye contact
- allowing time, not rushing and allowing periods of silence so that the information can be absorbed
- avoiding platitudes such as 'I know what you are going through'; rather reflect back on their emotions, e.g. 'It must be a terrible shock for you'
- answering questions in a sympathetic and non-judgemental way
- sharing a cup of tea (if appropriate) – this can help the relationship (Wright, 1996).

The family members may reach for physical contact, such as holding hands, or an arm around the shoulder, or they may withdraw, even avoiding eye contact.

It can also be a very emotional time for the staff involved, and family members are often grateful to see this. It can convey a message that their child was really cared for by staff members. Although some display of emotion should not be seen as unprofessional or a sign of weakness, it should not become a situation where the relatives are comforting the staff.

What to tell the family

The way bad news is broken is critical. Words like dead or died are unequivocal and will not be misinterpreted. Honest direct information about the sequence of events, from practitioners who do not skirt around the real issues, is valued by relatives (Wright, 1996).

The family should be told in plain language that the child has died despite all efforts to save his/her life. Phrases such as 'we've lost him', or 'she slipped away', or even 'passed on', can be misleading, or misinterpreted, leading to even more distress when the truth is finally realized (Morton and Phillips, 1996).

Telephone notification of the family members

Telephone notification of the family members can be difficult and is never easy. To minimize confusion and misunderstanding, the information should be clear and concise. The following is suggested:

- Identify yourself and the hospital.
- Establish who it is you are speaking to – if the person is not the key family member, find out where he or she can be contacted.
- Give the name of the child and ward. It seems to be common practice not to inform relatives over the telephone that the child has died, but instead to tell them that the child's condition has deteriorated rapidly, is critical, or words to that effect. A dilemma arises if the nurse is asked if the child has died. The author's view is that an honest approach is preferable. Wright (1996) suggests that if the hospital is easily accessible, relatives should be told when they arrive and not over the phone.
- Check that the family are clear about the message and are familiar with how to get to the hospital.
- Document the exact details of the telephone conversation.

Practical arrangements following a death

Cultural and religious requirements

As part of the family care and the last offices for the child, any specific religious or cultural requirements should be ascertained. It may be necessary to request a hospital chaplain, or a local religious leader to be present with the family and child. When a baby has died, the family may wish for him/her to be baptized and this should be arranged as quickly as possible (Huband and Trigg, 2000). It is useful to keep a list of contacts for the main religions, if the family are unable to provide specific details.

Expressions of grief and handling the body can vary depending on the patient's religion and cultural background. The *Nursing Times* 'Death With Dignity' booklets, which detail specific beliefs and procedures in the event of death for most religions, are very useful.

Viewing the child's body

Whilst the family are being informed about the death of their child, nursing staff can be preparing the child for viewing. In most cases, even for coroner's referrals, medical equipment such as tracheal tubes, intravenous cannulae, intraosseous needles can be removed, but it should be ascertained that this is appropriate before doing so. The child should have any obvious blood or other bodily fluids cleaned away, but a thorough wash is not usually necessary, and could potentially remove evidence for the Coroner. Any wounds should be covered with a dry dressing.

The child should be dressed in his or her own clothes if suitable, if not an appropriately sized gown or spare clothes – a shroud is never appropriate. Staff should ensure that the child is laid on and covered by clean sheets; the room should be private, without risk of intrusion. The child should be positioned supinely, and the eyes should be closed. A baby could be laid in a Moses basket, to look less clinical.

The family members should be informed of how their child appears before entering the room, especially if there are obvious injuries. Once in the room, they should be encouraged to hold their child (if able), talk to the child if they want to. This allows the grieving process to begin by accepting that their child is dead. Although the family must never be rushed through this, there has to come a time when they have to leave their child. There should be a protocol regarding how they can return to view their child, perhaps with other family members.

Role of the police and Coroner

The family should be made aware that the police and the Coroner will be informed, and that this is standard practice for all sudden unexplained paediatric deaths. If the child arrived via an emergency ambulance, then it is likely that the police will have picked up the call and would have already arrived. If not, then the senior doctor on duty is obliged to call them. Quite often the police will return to the address where the child was when he or she collapsed to collect evidence (Morton and Phillips, 1996). This can obviously be very distressing for the family. It is very important to emphasize that this is routine, and that the parents are not necessarily under suspicion of wrongdoing.

As with all sudden deaths, the doctor in charge of the child's care or the police will refer to the Coroner to decide whether a post-mortem examination is required. If the Coroner decides a post-mortem is required, the family cannot refuse, as this is a legal decision. But the family should be reassured as to what the examination will entail, that it will resolve the question as to why their child has died. It is very important that the relatives are told that great care is taken to retain the child's normal appearance, and that the family will be able to view the child again once the post-mortem has been performed.

As part of the Coroner's investigation, it may be necessary for the child to have certain investigations performed in the first few hours after death. This can include blood tests, urine collection, skin biopsy, skeletal survey X-rays. This is mainly to investigate natural causes of death, such as metabolic disease, or genetic disorders, but can also assist in determining any unnatural cause of death. It is essential that staff keep the clothes that the child was wearing, including the nappy if relevant. The police may take these items as evidence. If not, they should accompany the child to the mortuary, properly labelled.

Information for the family

It is essential that the family members are given written information regarding arrangements for their child (Fig. 12.1). At such a distressing

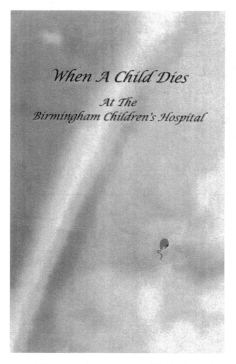

Fig. 12.1 Bereavement literature (reproduced with kind permission of Birmingham Children's Hospital, UK).

time, the family will not be able to remember verbal information, and this could lead to unnecessary confusion and added stress for them.

The information should include the name and telephone number of a nominated person, such as a bereavement counsellor, or a nominated nurse who can act as a central contact in the event of any queries, also the contact number for the Coroner's office, or police officer assigned to them. This advice should also contain information about who to contact should relatives wish to return to view the child.

It can also be useful to provide the names and telephone numbers of any agencies that can provide support, such as The Foundation for the Study of Infant Death, The Child Bereavement Trust or Child Death Helpline.

Keepsakes

Many areas offer the relatives a memorial booklet, containing such items as a lock of hair, a photograph, hand/footprints. It has been shown that such mementoes are well received by the family, but it should be at the discretion of the nurse caring for the family whether they are offered immediately, or given at a later time (Simons, 1998). It should be remembered if a Polaroid camera is used for photographs that they can fade over time, and this should be mentioned to the family.

Transport arrangements

The nurse caring for the family needs to make travel arrangements to take the relatives home; they should never be allowed to drive themselves.

Communication with other agencies

Other relevant agencies, e.g. general practitioner, health visitor and child's school, need to be informed about the child's death as soon as possible, as they may be able to provide support to family members.

Staff support

Dealing with the sudden death of a child is a very stressful event for all healthcare professionals. There may be a feeling that the team has 'failed' in its resuscitation attempts, or that perhaps they should have tried for longer. Being involved in the attempt to save a child's life is very emotional and distressing, and for that reason such resuscitations may be longer, owing to staff being unwilling to give up.

Due to the nature of the situation, it is vital that staff involved are offered the chance to debrief. This should be a formal process, facilitated by someone who has the appropriate training and skills required. Ideally it should include all members of the multidisciplinary team who were involved, and some centres invite pre-hospital personnel, such as paramedics. This can be the ideal time to raise questions about treatment or procedures, and receive reassurance about the outcome.

Before the family leave, it is vital that a thorough medical history of the events that led up to the child's death is taken. This could have been done whilst the family were waiting during the resuscitation, or it could be done afterwards. It is unlikely that parents will be able to remember specific details at a later time, and accurate record keeping is essential, especially if there were to be an inquest or criminal investigation (Advanced Life Support Group, 2001).

Importance of written guidelines and policies

The key to coping with such situations is to ensure that there are written guidelines and policies to follow. This should facilitate an organized plan of care for both the child and the family, and therefore minimize the distress for both the relatives and staff. Even if paediatric death is a very rare occurrence, to have such written information will be invaluable when dealing with an already fraught event.

Such guidelines and policies should be easily accessible; all staff should be encouraged to read them regularly, therefore keeping themselves up to date. It is easiest if they take the form of a flowchart, as they are organized and logical. All local protocols regarding Coroner referrals, contact telephone numbers, mortuary arrangements etc., should be stored with the hospital policies, therefore keeping all the necessary information and relevant paperwork together.

It can be helpful to have nominated staff members who are responsible for updating this information, and who could also be contact points for other agencies (police, Coroner etc.) when new policies or practices are being introduced.

Family members witnessing resuscitation

Being separated from a loved one, particularly at the time of death, can cause considerable distress (Renner, 1991). Should relatives therefore be present during resuscitation?

This issue has been extensively debated in the literature in recent years, most commonly in relation to adult resuscitation. Some practitioners believe that relatives should be allowed to witness resuscitation (Adams *et al.*, 1994). Others point out that having relatives present can cause anxiety for junior doctors, other staff and also for the relatives themselves, particularly if invasive procedures are being undertaken (Schilling, 1994; Zoltie *et al.*, 1994).

Advantages of family members witnessing resuscitation

There are a number of advantages of family members witnessing resuscitation. Witnessing the resuscitation:

- reinforces the fact that the child has died, avoiding prolonged denial and assisting with the bereavement process
- avoids distress that may have been brought on by being separated from the child

- enables the family members to talk to the child
- allows the family members to see for themselves that everything possible was done
- allows the family members to touch and speak with the deceased while the body is still warm (adapted from Resuscitation Council (UK), 2000a).

Disadvantages of family members witnessing resuscitation

Disadvantages of family members witnessing resuscitation include the possibility of:

- causing distress, particularly if invasive procedures are undertaken
- hindering the cardiac arrest team, physically or emotionally.

Necessary safeguards when family members witness resuscitation

If family members witness the resuscitation, it is vital that the allocated family nurse stays with them constantly, being able to explain procedures, answer questions, and observe for signs of them becoming overwhelmed with the situation (Huband and Trigg, 2000). It should be emphasized that they are able to leave the room at any time, or that they will be asked to leave if they are becoming too distressed, or interfere with the resuscitation attempt.

Summary

Dealing with the sudden death of a child can be deeply stressful for both staff and family members. Healthcare professionals need to know how to support bereaved family members through the process of grieving following a child's death. This chapter has discussed the principles of the early management of bereavement, including how to break bad news. Allowing family members to witness resuscitation can help with the bereavement process.

Chapter 13

Records, record keeping and audit

Introduction

An accurate written record detailing the paediatric resuscitation event is essential. It forms an integral part of the medical and nursing management of the child and can help to protect the practitioner if defence of his or her actions is required.

Unfortunately the exact timing and sequence of events and interventions can sometimes be difficult to recall. Nevertheless, despite this, accurate record keeping will still be expected. In addition audit of in-hospital resuscitation attempts should be on-going following national and international guidelines.

The aim of this chapter is to understand the principles of good record keeping and audit.

Objectives

At the end of the chapter the reader will be able to:

- discuss the importance of accurate record keeping
- outline the principles of effective record keeping
- detail what post-resuscitation records should include
- discuss the uniform reporting of data related to in-hospital resuscitation
- discuss when records become a legal document
- outline the National Audit of Paediatric Resuscitation (NAPR) study.

Importance of accurate record keeping

Accurate record keeping will help to protect the welfare of the child by promoting high standards of clinical care and continuity of care through better communication and dissemination of information between members of the interprofessional healthcare team. Accurate records will also help the practitioner to promptly detect any changes in the child's condition.

Principles of effective record keeping

According to the UKCC (now NMC) (1998) (Fig. 13.1), there are a number of factors which contribute to effective record keeping. The records should:

- be factual, consistent and accurate
- be documented as soon as possible after the event

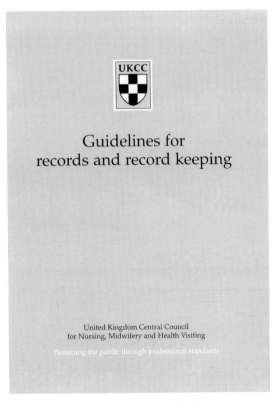

Fig. 13.1 Guidelines for records and record keeping (UKCC, 1998).

- provide current information on the care and condition of the patient
- be documented clearly and in such a way that the text can not be erased
- have any alterations and additions dated, timed and signed with all original entries clearly legible
- be accurately dated, timed and signed (including a printed signature)
- not include abbreviations, jargon, meaningless phrases, irrelevant speculation.

What post-resuscitation records should include

It is most important that the resuscitation attempt is fully documented in the notes. The following should be included:

- time of arrest, including presenting ECG rhythm
- events leading up to arrest
- details of resuscitation including ECG rhythms and response to treatment
- tracheal intubation time and duration of ventilation
- details of drugs administered, including doses and routes used

- details of defibrillation, particularly the time interval from the recognition of a shockable rhythm to the first shock
- any pertinent blood chemistry, e.g. arterial blood gases, pH and base deficit
- results
- names of personnel, including designation, present
- reasons for any delay in starting resuscitation
- details of communication with the parents
- when resuscitation was stopped, either because it was successful or because it was abandoned.

The clinical records should be legible and accurately reflect what happened during the resuscitation attempt. In addition, uniform reporting of data related to in-hospital resuscitation attempts will enable an accurate evaluation of the resuscitation attempt and provide an indication of the effectiveness of the European Resuscitation Council guidelines (2001).

Uniform reporting of data related to in-hospital resuscitation attempts

In order to evaluate the precise effectiveness of resuscitation and the European Resuscitation Council guidelines, it is important to produce robust scientific data on a national and international level.

The in-hospital Utstein style of data collection provides guidelines for the uniform reporting of data relating to in-hospital resuscitation attempts. The Utstein style identifies four distinct variables, which require data collection:

- hospital variables
- child variables
- event variables
- outcome variables.

At the time of writing, the Utstein template was being reviewed by the Resuscitation Council (UK).

Records as a legal document

There is often concern as to what constitutes a legal document. Basically any document requested by the court becomes a legal document (Dimond, 1994), e.g. nursing records, medical records, X-rays, laboratory reports, in fact any document which may be relevant to the case. If any of the documents are missing, the writer of the records may be cross-examined as to the circumstances of their disappearance (Dimond, 1994):

> Medical records are not proof of the truth of the facts stated in them but the maker of the records may be called to give evidence as to the truth as to what is contained in them.

National Audit of Paediatric Resuscitation (NAPR) study

The National Audit of Paediatric Resuscitation (NAPR) study is funded by the Resuscitation Council (UK) and coordinated by the Resuscitation Department at Hammersmith Hospital in London. Data are collected on paediatric resuscitation (excluding newborn resuscitation). It is hoped that the study will establish a central registry for all paediatric resuscitation events in the UK, and then hopefully throughout Europe.

The study is a retrospective audit of paediatric resuscitation procedures and outcomes when using the current Resuscitation Council (UK) guidelines for paediatric BLS and ALS. Collection of data began on January 1 2001 and will continue initially for a 2-year period. It is recommended to use the paediatric Utstein template for collecting data, which at the time of writing is under review.

For further information, access the Resuscitation Council (UK) website: http://www.resus.org.uk. To register for the project complete the registration form on the website and forward it to:

NAPR
C/o Dr David Zideman
Consultant Anaesthetist
Department of Anaesthetics
Hammersmith Hospital
Du Cane Road
London W12 OHS, UK

Summary

Accurate record keeping following a paediatric resuscitation is essential. The records must be:

- factual
- legible
- clear
- concise
- accurate
- signed, timed and dated.

Data from paediatric resuscitation attempts should be collected using the Utstein style of data collection. Participation in the NAPR study is encouraged.

Chapter 14

Ethical and legal issues

Introduction

When required, it is important to commence resuscitation promptly and effectively, following European Resuscitation Council guidelines (2001). It is also important to recognize when such measures should stop or should be withheld.

There are therefore a number of ethical and legal issues faced by practitioners who may be involved in providing CPR (BMA *et al.*, 2001). In the current NHS climate with the increasing risk of litigation, it is important for practitioners to ensure that they are always able to justify their actions and provide a reasonable standard of care.

The aim of this chapter is to provide an introduction to the ethical and legal issues related to CPR. Further reading is essential if a comprehensive understanding is required or if policies and procedures need to be formulated.

Objectives

At the end of this chapter the reader will be able to:

- discuss what is meant by a 'reasonable standard of care'
- discuss the issues related to 'do not attempt resuscitation' orders
- discuss the factors influencing the decision to stop CPR
- outline a risk management strategy related to CPR.

Standard of care

A healthcare practitioner, e.g. a registered nurse, owes a 'duty of care' to a patient requiring CPR and is therefore expected to provide a reasonable standard of care. Although at present there is no English precedent, it is quite possible, as has happened in the USA, that in the future children and their parents may win claims for compensation for injury sustained during a CPR attempt if clinical negligence can be proved.

The key issue considered by the courts, regarding clinical negligence litigation claims, is an expectation that the child should have received a reasonable standard of care. Such standards will become increasingly higher in line with the objectives of the Government and clinical governance.

When determining whether this standard of care has been breached during any aspect of CPR, the level of experience and expertise that the practitioner has or is expected to have, together with the circumstances, will be taken into account. 'A claim of inexperience or lack of training will not be successful as a defence in an allegation of negligence if a practitioner has been called upon only to work within the limits of his own expected competence' (Resuscitation Council (UK), 1998).

On the other hand, if an ' inexperienced practitioner is obliged to commence emergency treatment, but at the same time calls for specialist help, his lack of training will normally be a defence if his performance is suboptimal' (Resuscitation Council (UK), 1998).

In the above circumstances, practitioners should consider the availability of more skilled help and should exercise a cautious degree of intervention within the realms of their own skills and training. It is also important to mention here, that where an expert practitioner takes control of a CPR procedure and delegates tasks to more junior members of staff within that team, that practitioner will remain accountable for any suboptimal treatment delivered by the junior member of staff, if the same was outside the junior staff member's range of experience and training. However, where there is a reckless or negligent acceptance of a delegated task, there is a liability on the practitioner accepting the task when the result is harm to the child.

In order to ascertain whether there has been a breach of duty, demonstrated by a fall in the standard of care delivered to the patient, it is first of all necessary to establish exactly what standard should have been followed and whether the defendant's actions differed, if at all, from what was reasonable to expect (Dimond, 1994).

The European Resuscitation Council has set a standard of care with the publication of CPR guidelines (European Resuscitation Council, 2001). The courts are likely to expect medical and nursing staff to ensure that they perform CPR to this standard, within of course their capabilities and experience. 'It is important that practitioners should not take on responsibility beyond the level to which they have been trained' (Resuscitation Council (UK), 1998).

To determine the legal standard expected from practitioners, the courts apply the so-called Bolam test, which derives from a case decided in 1957. It was in the Bolam case that the standard was first described as when there is a:

> situation which involves the use of some special skill or competence, then the test as to whether there has been negligence or not is ... the standard of the ordinary skilled man exercising and professing to have that special skill. A man need not possess the highest expert skill; it is well established that it is sufficient if he exercises the ordinary skill of an ordinary competent man exercising that particular art.

It was also stated in the Bolam case that:

> 'a doctor is not negligent if he is acting in accordance with a practice accepted as proper by a reasonable body of medical men skilled in that art' and further he is not necessarily negligent 'merely because there is a body of such opinion that takes a contrary view.'

(The Bolam test applies to all healthcare professionals not just medical staff.)

Therefore, the approach a practitioner decides to adopt during CPR may not necessarily be negligent in all circumstances. However, deviating from nationally recognized guidelines would require clear explanation and justification as to why the guidelines did not apply in those particular circumstances, should the patient suffer harm as a result.

When considering guidelines and protocols for CPR, the practitioner must always consider the best interests of the child. If applying a standard method of treatment, supported by a protocol or guideline that is clearly not relevant to the child's needs, results in an adverse outcome for the child then the practitioner would be culpable under the Bolam principle.

In the *Airedale Hospitals NHS Trust* v *Bland* case (1993), the court found that the medical staff, who had followed the withdrawal of treatment guidelines published by the GMC, were not negligent because the guidelines satisfied the Bolam test. The judges took pains to point out that, had the guidelines not been in line with current accepted practice, the blind following of them would not have protected the Trust against a finding of negligence.

In the more recent case of *Bolitho* v *City and Hackney Hospital* (1998), the court considered the sensibility of the application of the Bolam test for the first time since 1957. The judges held that it could not simply be the case that, where there was support for a defendant doctor's actions through a responsible body of medical opinion, the doctor would not be negligent. The supporting opinion itself must be capable of logical analysis and commonsensical application.

For the Bolam test, this means that there is an additional criterion to a doctor not being negligent merely because there is a body of opinion with a contrary view. Whilst this is still true, the converse is that a doctor may still be negligent even if there is a body of medical opinion which takes a supportive view unless that body of opinion can convince the court that it is reasonable in all the circumstances.

According to Dimond (1994), there are a number of lessons to be learnt from court cases in relation to expected standards of care. Those that can be applied to CPR are as follows:

- The practitioner must be familiar with current standards of practice. This includes being aware of protocols, guidelines and procedures which have been drawn up locally and nationally, and keeping abreast of changes and updates.
- Despite the availability of guidelines, there is still room for professional judgement and discretion. However, clear and precise records need to be kept detailing the particular circumstances and justifications for departing from approved protocols and standards.
- The practitioner's knowledge and skills should be kept up to date because under clinical governance and Government initiatives for the improvement of healthcare, standards of care are likely to rise. The practitioner will be judged against the standard most universally applied at the time of the incident. In this context the practitioner should be aware

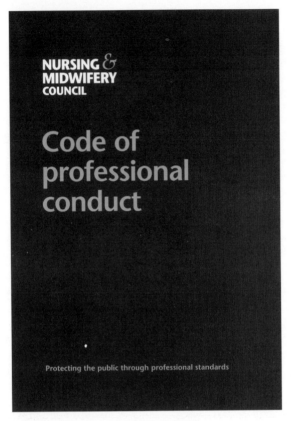

Fig. 14.1   *Code of professional conduct* (NMC, 2002).

that where there are conflicting standards, the courts will often prefer the one which was least likely to result in harm to the child.

An appropriate standard of care is also expected from the professional bodies. In the *Code of professional conduct* (NMC, 2002) (Fig. 14.1), it states that:

- 'in an emergency, in or outside the work setting, you have a professional duty to provide care. The care provided would be judged against what could be reasonably expected from someone with your knowledge, skills and abilities when placed in those particular circumstances'
- 'you have a responsibility to deliver care based on current evidence, best practice and, where applicable, validated research when it is available'.

Issues related to 'do not attempt resuscitation' orders

The main purpose of medical treatment is to benefit the child by restoring or maintaining health as far as possible, thereby maximizing benefit and minimizing harm. If treatment fails or ceases to be beneficial, it may not be in the best interests of the child to undertake CPR.

It is therefore important to identify any children for whom cardiac arrest represents a terminal event in their illness and in whom CPR is inappropriate. It is also important to identify any competent child who does not want CPR to be attempted and who competently refuses it.

When discussing a 'do not attempt resuscitation' (DNAR) order it is important to consider:

- the likely clinical outcome, including the chances of successfully restarting the child's heart and breathing, and the overall benefit achieved from a successful CPR
- the child's wishes – these are an essential element to the decision
- the child's human rights (see below)
- the parents' wishes.

The views of children and young people should be taken into account when considering a DNAR order (BMA *et al.*, 2001). Competent young people can consent to medical treatment and when they lack competence it is usually the parents who act on their behalf.

In England, Wales and Northern Ireland medical staff are not necessarily bound by refusals of treatment by young people, because the courts have ruled that consent from people with parental responsibility, or from the court itself, still allows medical staff to provide treatment (BMA *et al.*, 2001). In Scotland, however, it is probable that a competent young person's decision cannot be overridden by the courts or by those with parental responsibility (BMA, 2001).

If disagreement persists despite attempts to reach agreement, it is recommended to seek legal advice (BMA *et al.*, 2001). It must be stressed that medical staff do not have to bow to demands from parents to provide treatment contrary to their professional judgement, although they will often try to accommodate the parents' wishes as far as possible as long as they would still be acting in the best interests of the child (Resuscitation Council (UK), 2001).

The BMA, Resuscitation Council (UK) and the RCN have produced a model information leaflet (BMA, 2002) (Fig. 14.2), on which local information leaflets can be based.

The Human Rights Act 1998 and DNAR orders

The Human Rights Act 1998 incorporates the majority of the rights set out in the European Convention on Human Rights into UK law. In order to meet their obligations under the Act, health professionals must be able to demonstrate that their decisions are compatible with the human rights identified in the Articles of the Convention (BMA *et al.*, 2001). Provisions particularly relevant to DNAR orders include the right to:

- life (Article 2)
- be free from inhuman or degrading treatment (Article 3)

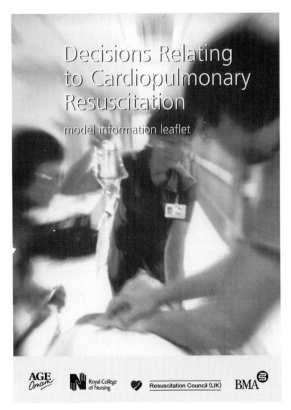

Fig. 14.2 Decisions relating to cardiopulmonary resuscitation: model information leaflet (BMA, 2002).

- respect for privacy and family life (Article 8)
- freedom of expression (Article 10)
- be free from discriminatory practices in respect of these rights (Article 14) (BMA *et al.*, 2001).

Who makes the decision?

It is widely recognized that any medical decisions relating to children and young people should ideally be taken within a supportive partnership involving them, their families and the healthcare team (BMA *et al.*, 2001).

The clinician in charge of the child's care is ultimately responsible for making a DNAR decision (BMA *et al.*, 2001). The views of other members of the healthcare team and the child's parents should also be sought. The views of children and young people should be taken into account when considering a DNAR order (BMA *et al.*, 2001).

Documentation

Once a DNAR order is made, 'not for attempted cardiopulmonary resuscitation' should be documented in the medical notes (BMA *et al.*, 2001). The entry should be signed and dated, and should include the rationale behind the order, who was consulted and when it should be reviewed.

The DNAR order should also be documented in the nursing notes by the primary nurse or most senior member of the nursing team, whose responsibility it is to communicate the decision to other members of the nursing team. Accurate record keeping is essential; it will help to protect the welfare of the child by promoting better communication and dissemination of information between members of the interprofessional healthcare team (UKCC, 1998).

Factors influencing the decision to stop CPR

Resuscitation is unlikely to be successful and can be discontinued if there has been no return of spontaneous circulation at any time with up to 30 minutes of cumulative CPR and in the absence of recurring or refractory VF/VT (ALSG, 2001). The child is unlikely to survive if there has been no return of spontaneous circulation despite two doses of adrenaline (epinephrine) (Young and Seidel, 1999). Prolonged CPR should be carried out if there is a history of poisoning or a primary hypothermia insult (American Heart Association, 2000).

Risk management strategy for CPR

'Professionals can take a risk management approach to litigation which on the one hand ensures high standards of care and on the other high standards of evidence should litigation be threatened' (Henderson and Jones, 1996).

Henderson and Jones (1996) have described the key components of a risk management strategy to minimize the risk of litigation:

• standards of care
• use of protocols
• monitoring practice
• identifying risk activities
• keeping records
• responding to complaints
• maintaining a safe environment.

Each is now discussed in turn in the context of infant and child resuscitation.

Standard of care

The law and the public will expect that the practitioner attains a recognized standard of care that would be expected from any competent healthcare professional. The practitioner will therefore need to keep up to date with current guidelines and strive to ensure that whenever possible practice is based on evidence. This will of course require not only knowledge but also, and certainly more importantly, competency at resuscitation skills. This is where, in particular, training and regular updates in CPR techniques are essential if this required level of competency is not only to be reached but also maintained.

There should also be an audit system in place to ensure that these standards are being achieved and maintained. One objective method of undertaking this is through scenario testing using a manikin, preferably in the clinical area, following Resuscitation Council (UK) guidelines. It is more beneficial if the team approach to CPR is evaluated and it is therefore desirable to encourage participation of the crash team members. This will help ensure a more realistic CPR situation.

Protocols

Protocols, e.g. who should attend a CPR attempt, can help to reduce the risk of error and help to ensure that the desired standard of care is delivered. Where appropriate, they should be based on current research, guidelines and recommendations and should be determined and agreed locally. It is important to ensure that all practitioners who will be expected to follow them are involved in their production. This will help to ensure that they are followed.

Monitoring practice

All CPR attempts should be audited (see Ch. 13). This can be done either by completing a standard audit form immediately following the event (preferable), or retrospectively by reviewing the child's notes. The main purpose of the audit is to identify any problems, e.g. with equipment or with the resuscitation procedure, and rectify them accordingly. In addition, potential problems may be highlighted.

Identifying risk activities

Risk activities should be identified, e.g. decisions on when to request senior medical support during CPR is one area of clinical practice which is prone to or favours successful litigation. It is important to ensure that regular training is undertaken and appropriate protocols are in place and regularly reviewed.

Keeping records

The keeping of clear comprehensive records is part of the duty of care owed to the patient (Dimond, 1994). In addition, they are invaluable when providing evidence in cases of litigation. It is therefore imperative to ensure that high standards of record keeping are maintained. *Guidelines for records and record keeping*, published by the UKCC (now NMC) (1998), provides guidance on this important subject (see Ch. 13).

Responding to complaints

Ideally complaints should be investigated and settled at an early stage. This will then hopefully prevent them from turning into formal complaints. In addition good communication and explanations may also reduce the incidence of complaints in the first place.

Maintaining a safe environment

The requirements of the Health and Safety at Work Act (1974) should be followed. Particular care should be taken with sharps and body fluids. Regular checks should be carried out on the CPR equipment, following the manufacturers' recommendations, and any faults or defects reported and rectified.

Summary

When required, it is important to commence resuscitation promptly and effectively following European Resuscitation Council guidelines (2001). It is also important to recognize when such measures should stop or should be withheld. In the current NHS climate, with increasing risks of litigation, it is important for practitioners to ensure that they are always able to justify their actions and provide a reasonable standard of care.

Chapter 15

Resuscitation training

Introduction

'Training in paediatric life support should be developed along flexible guidelines that will allow students to develop adequate and accurate skills in basic life support and advanced life support' (European Resuscitation Council, 1998). It is therefore essential to be able to provide realistic and lifelike training, particularly as paediatric cardiac arrests occur so infrequently and opportunities to gain practical experience in paediatric resuscitation are limited.

CPR employs skills that are essentially practical, and practitioners need hands-on practical training to both acquire and maintain them (*see* Resuscitation Council (UK), 2000d). The methods used to teach CPR techniques have been the subject of much investigation in recent years. Considerable effort has been devoted by teachers and educationalists to determining the optimum method of teaching CPR techniques, so that the necessary skills are both acquired and easily retained.

The aim of this chapter is to understand the principles of resuscitation training.

Objectives

At the end of the chapter the reader will be able to:

- discuss why resuscitation training is important
- outline the principles of adult learning
- describe the methods of resuscitation training
- state the key learning objectives of paediatric resuscitation training
- describe what training manikins and models are currently available for resuscitation training.

Why resuscitation training is important

Resuscitation training is important because:

- Practitioners' skills in resuscitation are often very poor (Lowenstein *et al.*, 1981; Wynne *et al.*, 1987; Buss *et al.*, 1993).
- There is considerable disparity between perceived competence and the actual ability to undertake effective resuscitation (Smith and Hatchett, 1992).
- The experience of senior practitioners attending cardiac arrests is that confidence levels are often high but this is generally not matched by high skill levels (Wynne *et al.*, 1987).

- Retention of CPR skills is very poor (McKenna and Glendon, 1985; Moser and Coleman, 1992); a significant deterioration in competence has been shown after only 10 weeks (Broomfield, 1996). At present there is unfortunately no consensus on the best way to overcome this problem nor on how often refresher training is required. Certainly the more frequent the updates the better, though realistically an annual one is probably the most achievable.

Principles of adult learning

Adults are usually well motivated to learn once they realize that the course content is relevant to them. Adults generally learn best when they are treated as adults and when their skills, experience and prior knowledge are recognized and utilized.

The teacher can facilitate adult learning in several ways:

- acting as a resource person and helper
- explaining points that have not been understood
- demonstrating principles, concepts and skills
- challenging the learner's values when appropriate
- adopting the role of task master and evaluator
- encouraging learner self-evaluation
- managing groups of learners effectively and facilitating the pursuit of intellectual questions (Fuszard, 1995).

Considerable research has been undertaken evaluating the principles of teaching basic and advanced CPR skills and factors affecting their retention. Both course content and time devoted to practice on manikins will influence skill attainment and subsequent retention of skills (Wynne, 1995).

Constructive feedback during training is important and should not only identify the student's strong points which will increase the student's confidence and motivation, but should also identify any weaknesses or deficiencies which need to be addressed and require more practice. In the event of poor performance, students should not be ridiculed.

Poor learner motivation, poor student–teacher relationship, physical and environmental factors all can create barriers to adult learning (Rogers, 1986).

Methods of resuscitation training

There are various methods of providing resuscitation training. The methods chosen will depend on a number of factors including time allocation, number of instructors, number of students, equipment, facilities and learning objectives. Quite often a variety of methods are used in each training session.

Regardless of the method used, it is recommended to adopt the following three-part approach to facilitate the teaching and learning process (Mackway-Jones and Walker, 1999):

Set   Ensure that the environment (lighting, heating, seating arrangements, audiovisual aids, training manikins, etc.) is adequate for training, set the mood, enhance the learners' motivation, state the session objectives and clarify the roles of the teacher and learners.

Dialogue (main teaching part of the session)   Ensure that the content is presented in a clear and logical format and at a level which the learners can understand; answer learners' questions appropriately and check learners have understood the content.

Closure   Include time for questions and queries from the learners, provide a concise summary and clearly terminate the session.

There are four key teaching methods that can be used in CPR training:

- lectures
- skill stations
- cardiac arrest scenarios
- discussion groups.

Lectures

Lectures can be used to revise core material, highlight key points and complement practical stations, but should not replace practical teaching on manikins and models. They also provide a valuable opportunity for group discussion. To help maintain interest, the lecturer should remember the following key points: conciseness, simplicity, eye contact, variations in speed and volume and the use of personal experience and questions (Mackway-Jones and Walker, 1999).

Skill stations (Fig. 15.1)

As CPR involves essentially practical skills, it is important to ensure that any training session allocates plenty of time for these skills to be taught and practised. Skill stations provide an opportunity to learn a skill and debate relevant issues. They should be placed in the context of the overall CPR procedure and be undertaken in small groups (ideally four to six persons). They should take into account, and build on, prior experience and knowledge of the students.

Shared aspects of teaching, learning and prior experience will promote both positive regard and mutual respect. Positive feedback, encouragement and guidance are also particularly important when teaching practical skills.

Mackway-Jones and Walker (1999) suggest a four-stage approach for teaching a practical skill.

Four-stage approach for teaching a practical skill
1. *The instructor demonstrates the skill at normal speed.* The skill is carried out at normal speed without explanation and commentary, except what

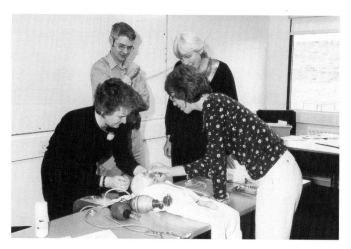

Fig. 15.1 Skill station.

would normally be said in the clinical situation. This allows the student to carefully observe the procedure without distraction.

2. *The instructor demonstrates the skill again, but this time with commentary.* The skill is demonstrated again, but this time with explanation. It will be broken down in small steps, and generally will not be at normal speed.

3. *The student provides the commentary while the instructor demonstrates the skill.* This stage is used because a skill is more likely to be learned if the student can describe it in detail. If the student is hesitant, the instructor can prompt by leading with the actions. On the other hand, confident candidates can describe the different stages of the skill before they are demonstrated. Any errors must be corrected immediately.

4. *The student demonstrates the skill together with commentary.* Each student then talks through and demonstrates the skill. The instructor now has an opportunity to observe each student to ensure that all individuals have understood, and are competent in, the skill.

Simulated cardiac arrest scenarios (Fig. 15.2)

Simulated cardiac arrest scenarios are a further method of teaching CPR skills. They can help to develop team work and help place CPR into context.

The scenarios, which should form a major part of any training session, follow on logically from the teaching and practice of individual skills, e.g. bag/valve/mask ventilation, chest compressions and intraosseous infusion. They are a way of putting it all together in a systematic and meaningful way. There are many advantages to this form of training:

- it is ideal for training in the clinical area
- it can help to effectively evaluate both an individual and a group performance (Kaye and Mancini, 1986)

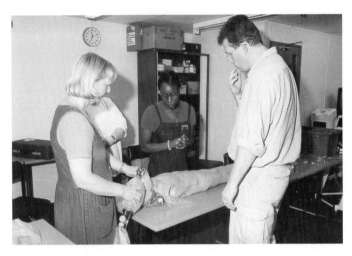

Fig. 15.2   Scenario teaching.

- it allows practitioners to practise their skills and to work as a team managing a paediatric 'cardiac arrest'
- it can help to bridge the theory/practice gap
- it can increase efficiency and credibility, improve communication and decision making and reduce anxiety (Wynne, 1995).

Discussion groups

Discussion groups, when well organized, are an effective teaching method (Resuscitation Council (UK), 2001d). Discussion reflects the method by which adults learn best, i.e. it is an active means of acquiring information (Mackway-Jones and Walker, 1999). Active group participation can result in an enjoyable learning experience (Abercrombie, 1989).

It is important to clearly define the desired outcome of the session, e.g. to reach a decision or consensus of opinion (convergent or closed discussion) or to facilitate learners to express and discuss their views (divergent or open discussion) (Resuscitation Council (UK), 2001d).

Resuscitation Council (UK) Paediatric Advanced Life Support (PALS) course

The main emphasis of the Resuscitation Council (UK) Paediatric Advanced Life Support (PALS) course is on the recognition of an infant or child in established respiratory or circulatory failure and the development of knowledge and skills required to prevent further deterioration towards cardiac arrest. The management of a paediatric arrest is also taught.

The course is run over 2 days and comprises lectures, skill stations, scenarios and assessments. A course manual is forwarded to the participants approximately 4 weeks prior to the start of the course. For further information contact the Resuscitation Council (UK) on 020 7388 4678.

European Paediatric Life Support course

The European Resuscitation Council is introducing a European Paediatric Life Support course. At the time of writing it is still in the planning stages. It is very similar to the PALS course and is being designed for multi-disciplinary groups.

It will emphasize the recognition and initial management of the infant/child at risk of acute deterioration, with treatment being based on physiology rather than diagnosis. The emphasis will be on interventions that are known to be effective.

A pilot course was run in July 2002 and it is anticipated that the course will be introduced to the UK in 2004, replacing the PALS course.

Advanced Paediatric Life Support (APLS) course

The Advanced Paediatric Life Support (APLS) course is overseen by the Advanced Life Support Group (ALSG) in Manchester. This very intense course, which covers cardiac, serious illness and trauma emergencies, is aimed at senior clinicians working regularly with sick children. In addition, some course centres run APLS courses with a nursing component, enabling senior nurses to attend the course as well.

The course is run over 3 days and comprises lectures, workshops, skill sessions, scenarios and assessments. A course manual is forwarded to the participants approximately 4 weeks prior to the start of the course. For further information contact the ALSG on 0161 877 1999.

Paediatric Life Support (PLS) course

The Paediatric Life Support (PLS) course is also overseen by the Advanced Life Support Group in Manchester. This popular course is aimed at nurses and medical staff who may be the first to respond in a paediatric emergency.

The course is run over 1 day and comprises lectures, workshops, skill sessions, scenarios and assessments. A course manual is forwarded to the participants approximately 4 weeks prior to the start of the course. For further information contact the ALSG on 0161 877 1999.

Key learning objectives of paediatric resuscitation training

Detailed below is a suggested list (not exhaustive) of key learning objectives which may help in the provision of CPR training. At the end of the session the learner will be able to:

- demonstrate the correct procedure for checking emergency equipment
- demonstrate the correct procedure for assessing a collapsed, apparently lifeless child

- state the correct procedure for summoning senior help
- demonstrate the correct procedure for opening and maintaining a clear airway, including use of suction
- demonstrate the correct procedure for insertion of an oropharyngeal airway
- demonstrate the correct procedure for bag/valve/mask ventilation and achieve chest rise on the manikin
- demonstrate effective chest compressions in both an infant and child on a manikin achieving a rate of 100 per minute
- describe and demonstrate the correct procedure for cricoid pressure
- list the equipment required for tracheal intubation
- list four complications of tracheal intubation
- demonstrate how to attach the cardiac monitor and select lead II
- demonstrate a safe technique for defibrillation in both an infant and a child
- list the hazards associated with defibrillation
- demonstrate the correct procedure for intraosseous infusion on a manikin
- specify the indications for administering adrenaline (epinephrine)
- discuss when CPR should be stopped.

Paediatric training manikins and models

Recent technological advances have enabled the manufacture of lifelike training manikins and models. These are transforming training because a greater number of clinical skills can now be demonstrated and practised in a controlled 'classroom' environment. A general overview of what is currently available is given below.

Airway management models (Fig. 15.3)

A number of infant and child airway management manikins are available. Most are anatomically correct in size and detail and benefit from having realistic landmarks including nostrils, tongue, oro- and nasopharynx, larynx, epiglottis, vocal cords, trachea, oesophagus, inflatable lungs and stomach.

Airway management skills that can be demonstrated and practised include the sizing and insertion of the oropharyngeal airway (Guedel airway), suction and tracheal intubation. However, it is not possible on some of the manikins to realistically perform facemask ventilation as the maintenance of an open airway is not always necessary to achieve chest rise. Laerdal's Resusci baby is a good manikin to practise this skill on because neutral position is required before chest rise can be achieved.

BLS manikins

Laerdal's Resusci Baby (Fig. 15.4) is claimed by the manufacturer to be 'the most realistic infant CPR manikin available'. Its features include natural airway obstruction where head tilt/chin lift is required to open the airway, and where over-extension of the neck will occlude it. An optional skill

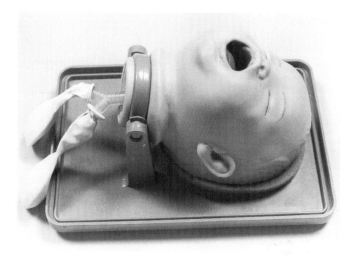

Fig. 15.3 Infant airway model (Laerdal).

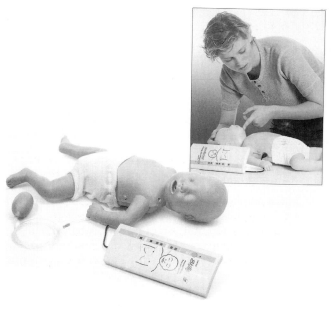

Fig. 15.4 Basic infant manikin (Laerdal).

guide provides objective feedback on ventilation and chest compression techniques and a brachial pulse simulator is a standard feature.

Resusci Junior (Laerdal) (Fig. 15.5) corresponds to a 5-year-old child. It benefits from realistic anatomical features and chest landmarks. A bilateral

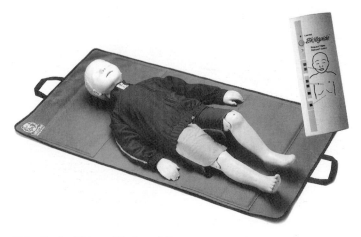

Fig. 15.5 Basic child manikin (Laerdal).

carotid pulse can be simulated. Optional extras include a skill guide providing objective feedback on CPR technique and a choking kit. In addition, a water rescue version is available. The manikin comes with a handy carrying case which opens out into a useful kneeling mat.

Also available are the basic low-cost infant and child manikins Baby Anne and Little Junior (Laerdal), which can be purchased individually or in a cost-saving pack of four. They allow more hands-on practice, which is particularly important when teaching paediatric CPR, as many find the techniques difficult to master and having to practise in front of colleagues can exacerbate the difficulty.

Intraosseous manikins

There are several intraosseous infusion manikins currently available that enable this life-saving skill to be demonstrated and practised. With some it is even possible to inject and aspirate fluid. Adam, Rouilly's infant intraosseous infusion simulator (Fig. 15.6), benefits from palpable key landmarks and enables students to practise the procedure with accuracy and realism.

ALS manikins

Multifunctional ALS manikins (Fig. 15.7) are ideal for training in team management of a paediatric cardiac arrest. Features generally include ECG monitoring, basic and advanced airway management including tracheal intubation, defibrillation, intraosseous infusion and drug administration as well as BLS. Practitioners can undertake tasks concurrently providing a more realistic and interactive training session.

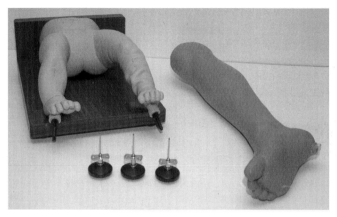

Fig. 15.6   Intraosseous models (Adam, Rouilly, left; Laerdal, right).

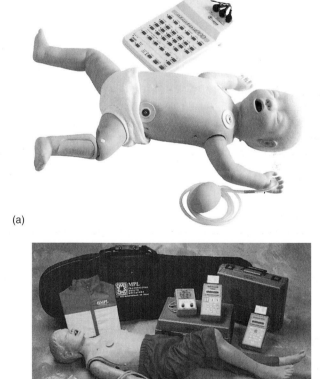

(a)

(b)

Fig. 15.7   (a) ALS infant, and (b) child manikins (Laerdal).

Manikin update kits

It is possible to update the older Resusci Baby and Resusci Junior models at a fraction of the cost of purchasing new ones. These manikin update kits, available from Laerdal, include the new and more convenient sanitation system – a disposable airway minimizes clean-up after class – and a removable face which can either be changed or disinfected between students. In addition, a new head undoubtedly improves the manikin's appearance.

Which manikin?

A number of factors need to be taken into account when purchasing a manikin, including number of staff to be trained and to what level, venue, storage, budget and power requirements. It is certainly recommended to see the manikin before purchasing it to ensure that it will meet your training requirements – some companies employ representatives to demonstrate their products, while others will offer them on a 'sale or return' basis. It is also advisable to seek advice from the local resuscitation training officer.

Maintenance of manikins

It is important to ensure that the manikins are properly maintained following the manufacturer's recommendations, particularly in relation to sanitation and the prevention of cross-infection (in addition seeking advice from an infection control nurse specialist is advisable).

Useful addresses

Training manikins are available from a number of companies including:

Laerdal Medical
Laerdal House
Goodmeade Road
Orpington
Kent BR6 0HX, UK
(Tel: 01689 876634)

Timesco of London
Timesco House
1 Knights Road
London E16 2AT, UK
(Tel: 020 7511 1234)

Summary

The importance of resuscitation training has been discussed. CPR skills are generally poor and regular training and retraining are required to ensure that competence and skills are maintained at a satisfactory level. The availability of lifelike manikins and models enables the provision of realistic resuscitation training.

References

Abercrombie, M. (1989) *The Anatomy of Judgement*. Free Association Books, London.

Abernethy, J. L., Allan, P. L. and Drummond, G. B. (1990) Ultrasound assessment of the position of the tongue during induction of anaesthesia. *Br. J. Anaesth.*, **65**, 744–748.

Adams, S., Whitlock, M., Higgs, R, *et al.* (1994) Should relatives be allowed to watch resuscitation? *BMJ*, **308**, 1687–1689.

Advanced Life Support Group (ALSG) (2001) *Advanced Paediatric Life Support: A Practical Approach*, 3rd edn. BMJ Books, London.

Airedale Hospitals NHS Trust v *Bland* [1993] 2 WLR 316.

American Academy of Pediatrics (1997) *Pediatric Advanced Life Support*. American Heart Association, USA.

American Academy of Pediatrics (2000) *Pediatric Education for Prehospital Professionals*. Jones & Bartlett, Sudbury USA.

American Academy of Pediatrics Committee on Drugs (1990) Naloxone dosage and route of administration for infants and children: addendum to emergency drug doses for infants and children. *Pediatrics*, **86**, 484–485.

American Heart Association (2000) *Guidelines 2000 for Cardiopulmonary Resuscitation and Emergency Cardiovascular Care*. American Heart Association, USA.

AHA and ILCOR (American Heart Association in Collaboration with ILCOR) (2000) Guidelines 2000 for cardiopulmonary resuscitation and emergency cardiovascular care – an international consensus on science. *Resuscitation*, **46**, 1–448.

Andersen, K. and Schultz-Lebahn, T. (1994) Oesophageal intubation can be undetected by auscultation of the chest. *Acta Anaesthesiol. Scand.*, **38**, 580–582.

Andropoulos, D. B., Soifer, S. J. and Schreiber, M. D. (1990) Plasma epinephrine concentrations after intraosseous and central venous injection during cardiopulmonary resuscitation in the lamb. *J. Pediatr.*, **116**, 312–315.

Atkins, D. L. and Kerber, R. L. (1992) Pediatric defibrillation: current flow is improved by using adult paddle electrodes. *Circulation*, **86(Suppl. 1)**, 1235.

Atkins, D., Sirna, S., Kieso, R. *et al.* (1988a) Pediatric defibrillation: importance of paddle size in determining transthoracic impedance. *Pediatrics*, **82**, 914–918.

Atkins, D., Hartley, L. and York, D. (1998b) Accurate recognition and effective treatment of ventricular fibrillation by automated external defibrillators in adolescents. *Pediatrics*, **101**, 393–397.

Aufderheide, T., Martin, D., Olson, D. *et al.* (1992) Prehospital bicarbonate use in cardiac arrest: a 3-year experience. *Am. J. Emerg. Med.*, **10**, 4–7.

Aydin, M., Baysal, K., Kucukoduk, S. *et al.* (1995) Application of ice water to the face in initial treatment of supraventricular tachycardia. *Turk. J. Pediatr.*, **37**, 15–17.

Bahr, J., Klingler, H., Panzer, W. *et al.* (1997) Skills of lay people in checking the carotid pulse. *Resuscitation*, **35**, 23–26.

Banai, S. and Tzivoni, D. (1993) Drug therapy for torsades de pointes. *J. Cardiovasc. Electrophysiol.*, **4**, 206–210.

Bardy, G. H., Ivey, T. D. and Allen, M. D. (1989) Evaluation of electrode polarity on defibrillation efficacy. *Am. J. Cardiol.*, **63**, 433–437.

Basket, P., Nolan, J. and Parr, M. (1996) Tidal volumes which are perceived to be adequate for resuscitation. *Resuscitation*, **3**, 231–234.

Beland, M., Hesslein, P., Finlay, C. *et al.* (1987) Non-invasive transcutaneous cardiac pacing in children. *PACE,* **10,** 1262–1270.

Bellingham, A., Detter, J. and Lenfant, C. (1971) Regulatory mechanisms of hemoglobin oxygen affinity in acidosis and alkalosis. *J. Clin. Invest.,* **50,** 700–706.

Berg, R. A. (1984) Emergency infusion of catecholamines into bone marrow. *Am. J. Dis. Child.,* **138,** 810.

Berg, M., Idris, A. and Berg, R. (1998) Severe ventilatory compromise due to gastric distension during pediatric cardiopulmonary resuscitation. *Resuscitation,* **36,** 71–73.

Bhende, M. and Thompson, A. (1995) Evaluation of an end-tidal CO_2 detector during pediatric cardiopulmonary resuscitation. *Pediatrics,* **95,** 395–399.

Bhende, M., Thompson, A., Cook, D. *et al.* (1992) Validity of a disposable end-tidal CO_2 detector in verifying endotracheal tube placement in infants and children. *Ann. Emerg. Med.,* **21,** 142–145.

Bingham, R. (1996) Cardiopulmonary resuscitation in children. In: *Cambridge Textbook of Accident and Emergency Medicine* (Skinner, D., Swain, A., Peyton, R. and Robertson, C. eds). Cambridge University Press, Cambridge.

Bintz, M. and Cogbill, T. (1996) Gastric rupture after the Heimlich manoeuvre. *J. Trauma,* **40,** 159–160.

Bishop, R. and Weisfeldt, M. (1976) Sodium bicarbonate administration during cardiac arrest: effect on arterial pH, PCO_2 and osmolality. *JAMA,* **235,** 506–509.

Bisogno, J., Langley, A. and Von Dreele, M. (1994) Effect of calcium to reverse the electrocardiographic effects of hyperkalaemia in the isolated rat heart: a prospective, dose-response study. *Crit. Care Med.,* **22,** 697–704.

Bjork, R., Snyder, B., Campion, B. *et al.* (1982) Medical complications of cardiopulmonary arrest. *Arch. Intern. Med.,* **142,** 500–503.

Bolitho v. *City and Hackney Health Authority* (HA) [1997] 3 WLR 1151.

Bowman, F., Menegazzi, J., Check, B. *et al.* (1995) Lower esophageal sphincter pressure during prolonged cardiac arrest and resuscitation. *Ann. Emerg. Med.,* **26,** 216–219.

Bradbury, N., Hyde, D. and Nolan, J. (2000) Reliability of ECG monitoring with a gel pad/paddle combination after defibrillation. *Resuscitation,* **44,** 203–206.

Brenner, B., Chavda, K., Karakurum, M. *et al.* (1999) Circadian differences among 4096 patients presenting to the emergency department with acute asthma. *Acad. Emerg. Med.,* **6,** 523.

Brenner, B., Kauffman, J. and Sachter, J. (1996) Comparison of the reluctance of house staff of metropolitan and suburban hospitals to perform mouth-to-mouth resuscitation. *Resuscitation,* **32,** 5–12.

British Association of A&E Medicine and Royal College of Nursing (1994) *Bereavement Care in A&E Departments.* RCN, London.

British Medical Association (BMA) (2001) *Consent, Rights and Choices in Health Care for Children and Young People.* BMJ Books, London.

British Medical Association (BMA) (2002) *Decisions Relating to Cardiopulmonary Resuscitation: Model Information Leaflet.* BMA, London.

British Medical Association (BMA), Resuscitation Council (UK) and the Royal College of Nursing (2001) *Decisions Relating to Cardiopulmonary Resuscitation: A Joint Statement.* BMA, London.

British Medical Association and Royal Pharmaceutical Society of Great Britain (2001) *British National Formulary.* BMA, London.

Broomfield, R. (1996) A quasi-experimental research to investigate the retention of basic cardiopulmonary resuscitation skills and knowledge by qualified nurses following a course in professional development. *J. Adv. Nurs.,* **23,** 1016–1023.

Brown, A. (1998) Therapeutic controversies in the management of acute anaphylaxis. *J. Accid. Emerg. Med.*, **15**, 89–95.

Burke, D. and Bowden, D. (1993) Modified paediatric resuscitation chart. *BMJ*, **306**, 1096–1098.

Bury Medical Unit (1994) *Audit of the Care of Bereaved Relatives Following Sudden Death.* 121 Silver Street, Bury BL9 OEN.

Buss, P., McCabe, M., Evans, R. *et al.* (1993) A survey of basic resuscitation knowledge among resident paediatricians. *Arch. Dis. Child.*, **68**, 75–78.

Cardenas-Rivero, N., Chernow, B., Stoiko, M. *et al.* (1989) Hypocalcaemia in critically ill children. *J. Pediatr.*, **114**, 946–951.

Carson, B. (1999) Successful resuscitation of a 44 year old man with hypothermia. *J. Emerg. Nurs.*, **25**, 5, 356–360.

Cavallaro, D. and Melker, R. (1983) Comparison of two techniques for detecting cardiac activity in infants. *Crit. Care Med.*, **11**, 189–190.

Cecchin, F., Perry, J., Berul, C. *et al.* (1999) Accuracy of automated external defibrillator analysis algorithm in young children. (Abstract) *Circulation*, **100(Suppl. 1)**, 663.

Ceneviva, G., Paschall, J., Maffei, F. *et al.* (1998) Hemodynamic support in fluid-refractory pediatric septic shock. *Pediatrics*, **102**, e19.

Cherian, L., Goodman, J. and Robertson, C. (1997) Hyperglycaemia increases brain injury caused by secondary ischaemia after cortical impact injury in rats. *Crit. Care Med.*, **25**, 1378–1383.

Clark, A. and Nasser, S. (2001) *Anaphylaxis Continuing Medical Focus: The State of Allergy/Immunotherapy in UK.* Rita Publications, London.

Cobbe, S., Redmond, M., Watson, J. *et al.* (1991) 'Heartstart Scotland'– initial experience of a national scheme for out of hospital defibrillation. *BMJ*, **302**, 1517–1520.

Colquhoun, M. and Camm, A. (1999) Asystole and electromechanical dissociation. In: *ABC of Resuscitation*, 4th edn (Colquhoun, M., Handley, A. and Evans, T. eds). BMJ Books, London.

Colquhoun, M. and Jevon, P. (2000) *Resuscitation in Primary Care.* Butterworth Heinemann, Oxford.

Connell, P., Ewy, G., Dahl, C. *et al.* (1973) Transthoracic impedance to defibrillation discharge: effect of electrode size and electrode–chestwall interface. *J. Electrocardiol.*, **6**, 313–317.

Cooper, M. (1995) Emergent care of lightning and electrical injuries. *Semin. Neurol.*, **15**, 268–278.

Cote, C. and Todres, I. (1990) The paediatric airway. In: *A Practice of Anaesthesia for Infants and Children*, 2nd edn (Cote, C., Ryan, J., Todres, I. and Groudsouzian, N. eds). WB Saunders, Philadelphia.

Cowan, M., Bardole, J. and Dlesk, A. (1987) Perforated stomach following the Heimlich maneuver. *Am. J. Emerg. Med.*, **5**, 121–122.

Cross, K., Tizard, J. and Trythall, D. (1957) The gaseous metabolism of the newborn infant. *Acta Paediatr.*, **46**, 265–285.

Curran, C., Dietrich, A., Bowman, M. *et al.* (1995) Pediatric cervical-spine immobilisation: achieving neutral position? *J. Trauma*, **39**, 729–732.

D'Alecy, L., Lundy, E., Barton, K. *et al.* (1986) Dextrose containing intravenous fluid impairs outcome and increases death after eight minutes of cardiac arrest and resuscitation in dogs. *Surgery*, **100**, 505–511.

Dauchot, P. and Gravenstein, J. (1971) Effects of atropine on the electrocardiogram in different age groups. *Clin. Pharmacol. Ther.*, **12**, 274–280.

David, R. (1988) Closed chest cardiac massage in the newborn infant. *Pediatrics*, **81**, 552–554.

Deakers, T., Reynolds, G., Stretton, M. *et al.* (1994) Cuffed endotracheal tubes in pediatric intensive care. *J. Pediatr.,* **125,** 57–62.

Dembofsky, C., Gibson, E., Nadkarni, V. *et al.* (1999) Assessment of infant cardio-pulmonary resuscitation rescue breathing technique: relationship of infant and caregiver facial measurements. *Pediatrics,* **103,** E17.

Department of Health (DoH) (1991) *Welfare of Children and Young People in Hospital.* HMSO, London.

Derlet, R., Albertson, T. and Tharratt, R. (1991) Lidocaine potentiation of cocaine toxicity. *Ann. Emerg. Med.,* **20,** 135–138.

Dieckmann, R. and Vardis, R. (1995) High-dose epinephrine in pediatric out-of-hospital cardiopulmonary arrest. *Pediatrics,* **99,** 403–408.

Dimond, B. (1994) *Legal Aspects of Nursing,* 2nd edn. Prentice Hall, London.

Dracup, K., Moser, D., Doering, L. *et al.* (1998) Comparison of cardiopulmonary resuscitation training methods for parents of infants at high risk for cardio-pulmonary arrest. *Ann. Emerg. Med.,* **32,** 170–177.

Dykes, E., Spence, L., Young, J. *et al.* (1989) Preventable pediatric trauma deaths in a metropolitan region. *J. Pediatr. Surg.,* **24,** 107–110.

Eberle, B., Dick, W. F., Schneider, T. *et al.* (1996) Checking the carotid pulse check: diagnostic accuracy of first responders in patients with and without a pulse. *Resuscitation,* **33,** 107–116.

Eisenberg, M., Bergner, L. and Hallstrom, A. (1983) Epidemiology of cardiac arrest and resuscitation in children. *Ann. Emerg. Med.,* **12,** 672–674.

Epperly, T. and Stewart, J. (1989) The physical effects of lightning injury. *J. Fam. Pract.,* **29,** 267–272.

Ettinger, P., Regan, T. and Olderwurtel, H. (1974) Hyperkalaemia, cardiac conduction and the electrocardiogram: a review. *Am. Heart J.,* **88,** 360–371.

European Resuscitation Council (1998) *European Resuscitation Council Guidelines for Resuscitation.* Elsevier, Oxford.

European Resuscitation Council (2001) Guidelines 2000 for adult and paediatric basic life support and advanced life support. *Resuscitation,* **48,** 139–199.

Ewan, P. (1998) ABC of allergies: anaphylaxis. *BMJ,* **316,** 1442.

Ewan, P. and Clark, A. (2001) Long-term prospective observational study of patients with peanut and nut allergy after participation in a management plan. *Lancet,* **357,** 111.

Field, D., Milner, A. and Hipkin, I. (1986) Efficiency of manual resuscitators at birth. *Arch. Dis. Child.,* **61,** 300–302.

Finer, N., Barrington, K., Al-Fadley, F. *et al.* (1986) Limitations of self-inflating resus-citators. *Pediatrics,* **77,** 417–420.

Fiocchi, A., Restani, P., Ballabio, C. *et al.* (2001) Severe anaphylaxis induced by latex as a contaminant of plastic balls in play pits. *J. Allergy Clin. Immunol.,* **108(2),** 298–300.

Fiser, R., Walker, T., Seibert, J. *et al.* (1997) Tibial length following intraosseous infu-sion: a prospective, radiographic analysis. *Pediatr. Emerg. Care,* **13,** 186–188.

Fisher, M. (1986) Clinical observations on the pathophysiology and treatment of anaphylactic cardiovascular collapse. *Anaesth. Intensive Care,* **14,** 17–21.

Fisher, M. (1995) Treatment of acute anaphylaxis. *BMJ,* **311,** 731–733.

Flesche, C. W., Brewer, S., Mandel, L. P. *et al.* (1994) The ability of health profession-als to check the carotid pulse. *Circulation,* **90,** 282–288.

Fontanarosa, P. (1993) Electric shock and lightning strike. *Ann. Emerg. Med.,* **22(2),** 378–387.

Friedman, F. (1996) Intraosseous adenosine for the termination of supraventricular tachycardia in an infant. *Ann. Emerg. Med.,* **28,** 356–358.

Friesen, R. M., Duncan, P. and Tweed, W. (1982) Appraisal of pediatric cardio-pulmonary resuscitation. *Can. Med. Assoc. J.,* **126,** 1055–1058.

Fuchs, S., LaCovey, D. and Paris, P. (1991) A prehospital model of intraosseous infusion. *Ann. Emerg. Med.,* **20,** 371–374.

Fuszard, B. (1995) *Innovative Teaching Strategies in Nursing.* Aspen, Gaithersburg.

Geddes, L., Bourland, J. and Ford, G. (1986) The mechanism underlying sudden death from electric shock. *Med. Instrum.,* **20,** 303–315.

Gibbs, W., Eisenberg, M. and Damon, S. (1990) Dangers of defibrillation: injuries to personnel during patient resuscitation. *Am. J. Emerg. Med.,* **8,** 101–104 .

Gillis, J., Dickson, D., Reider, M. *et al.* (1986) Results of in-patient pediatric resuscitation. *Crit. Care Med.,* **14,** 469–471.

Glaeser, P. W. and Losek, J. D. (1986) Emergency intraosseous infusions in children. *Am. J. Emerg. Med.,* **4,** 34–36.

Glaeser, P. W., Losek, J. D. and Nelson, D. B. (1988) Pediatric intraosseous infusions: impact on vascular access time. *Am. J. Emerg. Med.,* **6,** 330–332.

Green, J. (1991) *Death with Dignity,* Vol. 1. Emap Healthcare, London.

Haley, C., McDonald, R., Rossi, L. *et al.* (1989) Tuberculosis epidemic among hospital personnel. *Infect. Control Hosp. Epidemiol.,* **10,** 204–210.

Handley, A. (1999) Basic life support. In: *ABC of Resuscitation,* 4th edn (Colquhoun, M., Handley, A. and Evans, T. eds). BMJ Books, London.

Handley, A. and Handley, J. (1995) The relationship between the rate of chest compression and compression : relaxation ratio. *Resuscitation,* **30,** 237–241.

Harrison, R. R. and Maull, K. I. (1982) Pocket mask ventilation: a superior method of acute airway management. *Ann. Emerg. Med.,* **11,** 74–76.

Hartrey, R. and Bingham, R. (1995) Pharyngeal trauma as a result of blind finger sweeps in the choking child. *Am. J. Emerg. Med.,* **12,** 52–54.

Hartrey, R. and Kestin, I. (1995) Movement of oral and nasal tracheal tubes as a result of changes in head and neck position. *Anaesthesia,* **50,** 682–687.

Hartsilver, E. and Vanner, R. (2000) Airway obstruction with cricoid pressure. *Anaesthesia,* **55,** 208–211.

Hazinski, M. F. (1995) Is paediatric resuscitation unique? Relative merits of early CPR and ventilation versus early defibrillation for young victims of cardiac arrest. *Ann. Emerg. Med.,* **25,** 540–543.

Hazinski, M., Walker, C., Smith, H. *et al.* (1997) Specificity of automated external defibrillator rhythm analysis in pediatric tachyarrhythmias. *Circulation,* **96(Suppl. 1),** 561.

Health and Safety at Work Act 1974. HMSO, London.

Heinild, S., Sodergaard, T. and Tudvad, F. (1974) Bone marrow infusions in childhood: experiences of 1000 infusions. *J. Pediatr.,* **30,** 400–412.

Henderson, C. and Jones, K. (1996) *Essential Midwifery.* Mosby, London.

Henning, R. (1992) Emergency transport of critically ill children: stabilisation before departure. *Med. J. Aust.,* **156,** 117–124.

Hess, D., and Baran, C. (1985) Ventilatory volumes using mouth to mouth, mouth to mask and bag/valve/mask techniques. *Am. J. Emerg. Med.,* **3,** 292–296.

Hirschman, A. and Kravath, R. (1982) Venting vs. ventilating: a danger of manual resuscitation bags. *Chest,* **82,** 369–370.

Hoffman, J., Votey, S., Bayer, M. *et al.* (1993) Effect of hypertonic sodium bicarbonate in the treatment of moderate-to-severe cyclic antidepressant overdose. *Am. J. Emerg. Med.,* **11,** 336–341.

Holzer, M., Behringer, W., Schorkhuber, W. *et al.* (1997) Hypothermia for Cardiac Arrest (HACA) Study Group, mild hypothermia and outcome after CPR. *Acta Anaesthesiol. Scand. Suppl.,* **111,** 55–58.

Homma, S., Gillam, L. and Weyman, A. (1990) Echocardiographic observations in survivors of acute electrical injury. *Chest,* **97,** 103–105.

Howard, R. and Bingham, R. (1990) Endotracheal vs. intravenous administration of atropine. *Arch. Dis. Child.,* **65,** 449–450.

Huang, Y., Wong, K., Yip, W. *et al.* (1995) Cardiovascular responses to graded doses of three catecholamines during lactic and hydrochloric acidosis in dogs. *Br. J. Anaesth.,* **74,** 583–590.

Huband, S. and Trigg, E. (eds) (2000) *Practices in Children's Nursing.* Churchill Livingstone, Edinburgh.

Hudgel, D. W. and Hendricks, C. (1988) Palate and hypopharynx: sites of inspiratory narrowing of the upper airway during sleep. *Am. Rev. Respir. Dis.,* **138,** 1542–1547.

Human Rights Act 1998. HMSO, London.

Idris, A., Wenzel, V., Banner, M. *et al.* (1995) Smaller tidal volumes minimise gastric inflation during CPR with an unprotected airway. (Abstract) *Circulation,* **92(Suppl 1),** 1759.

Idris, A. H., Florete, O. G. Jr., Melker, R. J. *et al.* (1996) Physiology of ventilation, oxygenation and carbon dioxide elimination during cardiac arrest. In: *Cardiac Arrest: The Science and Practice of Resuscitation Medicine* (Paradis, N. A., Halperin, H. R. and Nowak, R. M. eds). Williams & Wilkins, London.

Innes, P., Summers, C., Boyd, I. *et al.* (1993) Audit of paediatric cardiopulmonary resuscitation. *Arch. Dis. Child.,* **68,** 487–491.

Jasani, M., Nadkarni, V., Finkelstein, M. *et al.* (1994) Endotracheal epinephrine administration technique effects in pediatric porcine hypoxic–hypercarbic arrest. *Crit. Care Med.,* **22,** 1174–1180.

Jesudian, M. C., Harrison, R. R., Keenan, R. L. *et al.* (1985) Bag–valve–mask ventilation: two rescuers are better than one: preliminary report. *Crit. Care Med.,* **13,** 122–123.

Jevon, P. (2002) *Advanced Cardiac Life Support.* Butterworth-Heinemann, Oxford.

Jevon, P. and Ewens, B. (2002) *Monitoring the Critically Ill Patient.* Blackwell Science, Oxford.

Joglar, J., Kessler, D., Welch, P. *et al.* (1999) Effects of repeated electrical defibrillations on cardiac troponin I levels. *Am. J. Cardiol.,* **83(2),** (270–272), A6.

Johnson, L., Kissoon, N., Fiallos, M. *et al.* (1999) Use of intraosseous blood to access blood chemistries and hemoglobin during cardiopulmonary resuscitation with drug infusions. *Crit. Care Med.,* **27,** 1147–1152.

Johnston, C. (1992) Endotracheal drug delivery. *Pediatr. Emerg. Care,* **8,** 94–97.

Joly, H. R. and Weil, M. H. (1969) Temperature of the great toe as an indication of the severity of shock. *Circulation,* **39,** 131–138.

Kabbani, M. and Goodwin, S. (1995) Traumatic epiglottis following blind finger sweep to remove a pharyngeal foreign body. *Clin. Pediatr.,* **34,** 495–497.

Kaye, W. and Mancini, M. (1986) Use of the Mega Code to evaluate team leader performance during advanced cardiac life support. *Crit. Care Med.,* **14,** 99–104.

Kelly, M., Ewens, B. and Jevon, P. (2001) Hypothermia management. *Nurs. Times,* **97(9),** 36–37.

Kerber, R., Grayzel, L., Kennedy, J. *et al.* (1981) Elective cardioversion: influence of paddle electrode location and size on success rates and energy requirements. *N. Eng. J. Med.,* **305,** 658–662.

Kewalramani, L., Kraus, J. and Sterling, H. (1980) Acute spinal-cord lesions in a pediatric population: epidemiological and clinical features. *Paraplegia,* **18,** 206–219.

Khine, H., Cordrry, D., Kettrick, R. *et al.* (1997) Comparison of cuffed and uncuffed endotracheal tubes in young children in general anaesthesia. *Anesthesiology,* **86,** 627–631.

Kleinman, M., Oh, W. and Stonestreet, B. (1999) Comparison of intravenous and endotracheal epinephrine during electromechanical dissociation with CPR in dogs. *Ann. Emerg. Med.,* **27,** 2748–2754.

Klitzener, T. (1995) Sudden cardiac death in children. *Circulation,* **82,** 629–632.

Laerdal (1997) *Laerdal Silicone Resuscitators, Directions for Use.* Laerdal, Orpington, Kent.

La Fleche, F., Slepin, M., Vargas, J. *et al.* (1989) Iatrogenic bilateral tibial fractures after intraosseous infusion attempts in a 3 month old infant. *Ann. Emerg. Med.,* **18,** 1099–1101.

Langelle, A., Sunde, K., Wik, L. *et al.* (2000) Airway pressure with chest compressions versus Heimlich manoeuvre in recently dead adults with complete airway obstruction. *Resuscitation,* **44,** 105–108.

Larach, M. (1995) Accidental hypothermia. *Lancet,* **345,** 493–498.

Larsen, M., Eisenberg, M., Cummins, R. *et al.* (1993) Predicting survival from out-of-hospital cardiac arrest: a graphic model. *Ann. Emerg. Med.,* **22,** 1652–1658.

Lawes, E. G. and Baskett, P. J. F. (1987) Pulmonary aspiration during unsuccessful resuscitation. *Intens. Care Med.,* **13,** 379–382.

Lawrence, P. J. and Sivaneswaran, N. (1985) Ventilation during cardiopulmonary resuscitation: which method? *Med. J. Austr.,* **143,** 443–446.

Lee, P., Chung, Y., Lee, B. *et al.* (1989) The optimal dose of atropine via the endotracheal route. *Acta Anaesthesiol. Sin.,* **27(1),** 35–38.

Lermann, B. and Deale, O. (1990) Relationship between transcardiac and transthoracic current during defibrillation in humans. *Circ. Res.,* **67,** 1420–1426.

Levy, M. (1998) An evidence-based evaluation of the use of sodium bicarbonate during cardiopulmonary resuscitation. *Crit. Care Med.,* **14,** 457–483.

Lewis, J., Minter, M., Eshelman, S. *et al* (1983) Outcome of paediatric resuscitation. *Ann. Emerg. Med.,* **12,** 297–299.

Lim, S., Anantharaman, V., Teo, W. *et al.* (1998) Comparison of treatment of supraventricular tachycardia by Valsalva maneuver and carotid sinus massage. *Ann. Emerg. Med.,* **31,** 30–35.

Losek, J., Endom, E., Dietrich, A. *et al.* (1999) Adenosine and pediatric supraventricular tachycardia in the emergency department: multicenter study and review. *Ann. Emerg. Med.,* **33,** 185–191.

Lowenenstein, S., Libby, L., Mountain, R. *et al.* (1981) Cardiopulmonary resuscitation skills of medical and surgical house officers. *Lancet,* **2,** 679–681.

Lown, B. (1967) Electrical reversion of cardiac arrhythmias. *Br. Heart J.,* **29,** 469–489.

Lucking, S., Pollack, M. and Fields, A. (1986) Shock following generalised hypoxic–ischaemic injury in previously healthy infants and children. *J. Pediatr.,* **108,** 359–364.

Luten, R., Wears, R., Broselow, J. *et al.* (1992) Length-based endotracheal tube and emergency equipment in pediatrics. *Ann. Emerg. Med.,* **21,** 900–904.

McCabe, J., Cobaugh, D., Menegazzi, J. *et al.* (1998) Experimental tricyclic antidepressant toxicity: a randomised, controlled comparison of hypertonic saline solution, sodium bicarbonate and hyperventilation. *Ann. Emerg. Med.,* **32,** 329–333.

McKenna, S. and Glendon, A. (1985) Occupational first aid training. Decay in CPR skills. *J. Occup. Psychol.,* **58,** 109–117.

McKoy, C. and Bell, M. (1983) Preventable traumatic deaths in children. *J. Pediatr. Surg.,* **18,** 505–508.

Mackway-Jones, K. and Walker, M. (1999) *Pocket Guide to Teaching Medical Instructors*. BMJ Books, London.

McNamara, R. M., Spivey, W. H., Unger, H. D. *et al.* (1987) Emergency applications of intraosseous infusion. *J. Emerg. Med.*, **5**, 97–101.

Maier, G., Tyson, G. Jr., Olsen, C. *et al.* (1984) The physiology of external cardiac massage: high impulse cardiopulmonary resuscitation. *Circulation*, **70**, 86–101.

Majumdar, A. and Sedman, P. (1998) Gastric rupture secondary to successful Heimlich manoeuvre. *Postgrad. Med. J.*, **74**, 609–610.

Manolios, N. and Mackie, I. (1988) Drowning and near drowning on Australian beaches patrolled by life-savers: a 10-year study 1973–1983. *Med. J. Austr.* **148**, 170–171.

Mansell, A., Bryan, C. and Levison, H. (1972) Airway closure in children. *J. Appl. Physiol.*, **33**, 711–714.

Mather, C. and O'Kelly, S. (1996) The palpation of pulses. *Anaesthesia*, **51**, 189–191.

Matsumoto, T., Goto, Y. and Mike, T. (2001) Anaphylaxis to mite-contaminated flour. *Allergy*, **56(3)**, 247.

Mehta, S. (1990) A supraglottic oropharyngeal airway. *Anaesthesia*, **45**, 893–894.

Mejicano, G. and Maki, D. (1998) Infections acquired during cardiopulmonary resuscitation: estimating the risk and defining strategies for prevention. *Ann. Intern. Med.*, **129**, 813–828.

Melker, R. J. (1985) Recommendations for ventilation during cardiopulmonary resuscitation: a time for change? *Crit. Care Med.*, **13(Pt 2)**, 882–883.

Meltzer, L. *et al.* (1983) *Intensive Coronary Care: A Manual for Nurses*. Prentice Hall, London.

Molfino, N., Nannani, A., Matelli, A. *et al.* (1991) Respiratory arrest in near fatal asthma. *N. Eng. J. Med.*, **99**, 358–362.

Morton, R. and Phillips, B. (1996) *Accidents and Emergencies in Children*. Oxford University Press, Oxford.

Moser, D. and Coleman, S. (1992) Recommendations for improving cardio-pulmonary resuscitation skills retention. *Heart Lung*, **21**, 372–380.

Moynihan, R., Brock-Utne, J., Archer, J. *et al.* (1993) The effect of cricoid pressure on preventing gastric inflation in infants and children. *Anesthesiology*, **78**, 652–656.

Muzzi, D., Lossaso, T. and Cucchaira, R. (1991) Complication from a nasopharyn-geal airway in a patient with a basilar skull fracture. *Anesthesiology*, **74**, 366–368.

Nakakimura, K., Fleischer, J., Drummond, J. *et al.* (1990) Glucose administration before cardiac arrest worsens neurological outcome in cats. *Anesthesiology*, **72**, 1005–1011.

Nelson, L. and Hoffman, R. (1996) Toxicologic sudden death. In: *Cardiac Arrest: The Science and Practice of Resuscitation Medicine* (Paradis, N., Halperin, H. and Nowak, J. eds). Williams & Wilkins, London.

Noc, M., Weil, M., Sus, S. *et al.* (1994) Spontaneous gasping during cardio-pulmonary resuscitation without mechanical ventilation. *Am. J. Respir. Crit. Care Med.*, **150**, 861–864.

Nolan, J. P. and Parr, M. J. A. (1997) Aspects of resuscitation in trauma. *Br. J. Anaesth.*, **79**, 226–240.

Nursing and Midwifery Council (NMC) (2002) *Code of Professional Conduct*. NMC, London.

Oakley, P. (1988) Inaccuracy and delay in decision making in paediatric resuscita-tion and a proposed reference chart to reduce error. *BMJ*, **297**, 817–819.

Oakley, P. and Redmond, A. (1999) Post-resuscitation care. In: *ABC of Resuscitation*, 4th edn (Colquhoun, M., Handley, A. and Evans, T. eds). BMJ Books, London.

Oakley, P., Phillips, B., Molyneux, E. *et al.* (1993) Paediatric resuscitation. *BMJ,* **306,** 1613.

Orlowski, J. P. (1984) Optimal position for external cardiac massage in infants and children. *Crit. Care Med.,* **12,** 224.

O'Rourke, P. (1986) Outcome of children who are apnoeic and pulseless in the emergency room. *Crit. Care Med.,* **14,** 466–468.

Osterwalder, J. (1996) Naloxone: for intoxications with intravenous heroin and heroin mixtures: harmless or hazardous? *J. Toxicol. Clin. Toxicol.,* **34,** 409–416.

Otto, C., Yakaitis, R. and Blitt, C. (1981) Mechanism of action of epinephrine in resuscitation from asphyxial arrest. *Crit. Care Med.,* **9,** 321–324.

Overholt, E., Rheuban, K., Gutgesell, H. *et al.* (1988) Usefulness of adenosine for arrhythmias in infants and children. *Am. J. Cardiol.,* **61,** 336–340.

Paediatric Intensive Care Society (PICS) (2001) *Standards Document.* Paediatric Intensive Care Society.

Palme, C., Nystrom, B., Tunell, R. (1985) An evaluation of the efficiency of face masks in the resuscitation of newborn infants. *Lancet,* **1,** 207–210.

Paradis, N., Martin, G., Goetting, M. *et al.* (1989) Simultaneous aortic, jugular bulb, and right atrial pressures during cardiopulmonary resuscitation in humans: insights into mechanisms. (Abstract) *Circulation,* **80(Suppl 2).**

Patel, L., Radivan, F. and David, T. (1994) Management of anaphylactic reactions to food. *Arch. Dis. Child.,* **71,** 370–375.

Perez, A. (1996) Cardiac monitoring: mastering the essentials. *RN,* **59,** 32–39.

Petito, S. and Russell, W. (1988) The prevention of gastric inflation: a neglected benefit of cricoid pressure. *Anaesth. Intensive Care,* **16,** 139–143.

Phillips, G. W. and Zideman, D. A. (1986) Relation of infant heart to sternum: its significance in cardiopulmonary resuscitation. *Lancet,* **1,** 1024–1025.

Piazza, M., Chirianni, A., Picciotto, L. *et al.* (1989) Passionate kissing and micro-lesions of the oral mucosa: possible role in AIDS transmission. (Letter) *JAMA,* **261,** 244–245.

Poets, C., Meny, R., Chobanian, M. *et al.* (1999) Gasping and other cardiorespiratory patterns during sudden infant deaths. *Pediatr. Res.,* **45,** 350–354.

Project Team of the Resuscitation Council (UK) (1999) The emergency medical treatment of anaphylactic reactions. *J. Accid. Emerg. Med.,* **16(4),** 243–247.

Project Team of the Resuscitation Council (UK) (2001) Update on the emergency medical treatment of anaphylactic reactions for first medical responders and for community nurses. *Resuscitation,* **48,** 241–243.

Pulsineli, W., Waldman, S., Rawlinson, D. *et al.* (1982) Moderate hyperglycaemia augments ischaemic brain damage: neuropathologic study in the rat. *Neurology,* **32,** 1239–1246.

Quan, L. and Kinder, D. (1992) Pediatric submersions: prehospital predictors of outcome. *Pediatrics,* **90,** 909–913.

Quan, L., Graves, J., Kinder, D. *et al.* (1992) Transcutaneous cardiac pacing in the treatment of out-of-hospital pediatric cardiac arrests. *Ann. Emerg. Med.,* **21,** 905–909.

Quan, L., Wentz, K., Gore, E. and Copass, M. (1990) Outcome and predictors of outcome in pediatric submersion victims receiving pre-hospital care in King County, Washington. *Pediatrics,* **86,** 586–593.

Rattrie, E. (2000) Witnessed resuscitation: good practice or not? *Nurs. Stand.,* **14(24),** 32–35.

Renner, S. (1991) I desperately wanted to see my son. *BMJ,* **302,** 356.

Resuscitation Council (UK) (1998) *Advanced Life Support Provider Manual,* 3rd edn. Resuscitation Council (UK), London.

Resuscitation Council (UK) (2000a) *Advanced Life Support Provider Manual,* 4th edn. Resuscitation Council (UK), London.

Resuscitation Council (UK) (2000b) *Cardiopulmonary Resuscitation: Guidance for Clinical Practice and Training in Hospitals.* Resuscitation Council (UK), London.

Resuscitation Council (UK) (2000c) *Resuscitation Guidelines 2000.* Resuscitation Council (UK), London.

Resuscitation Council (UK) (2000d) *Generic Instructor Course: Advanced Life Support Instructor Manual.* Resuscitation Council (UK), London.

Resuscitation Council (UK) (2001) *Safer Handling during Resuscitation in Hospitals.* Resuscitation Council (UK), London.

Reuler, J. (1978) Hypothermia: pathophysiology, clinical settings and management. *Ann. Intern. Med.,* **89,** 519–527.

Rogers, A. (1986) *Teaching Adults.* Open University Press, Milton Keynes.

Rosen, P., Stoto, M. and Harley, J. (1995) The use of the Heimlich maneuver in near drowning: Institute of Medicine report. *J. Emerg. Med.,* **13,** 397–405.

Rosetti, V., Thompson, B., Aprahamian, C. *et al.* (1984) Difficulty and delay in intravenous access in pediatric arrests. *Ann. Emerg. Med.,* **13,** 406.

Rosetti, V., Thompson, B., Miller, J. *et al.* (1985) Intraosseous infusion: an alternative route of pediatric intravascular access. *Ann. Emerg. Med.,* **14,** 885–888.

Rosovsky, M., FitzPatrick, M., Goldfarb, C. *et al.* (1994) Bilateral osteomyelitis due to intraosseous infusion: case report and review of the English-language literature. *Pediatr. Radiol.,* **24,** 72–73.

Roth, B., Magnusson, J., Joahansson, I. *et al.* (1998) Jaw lift: a simple and effective method to open the airway in children. *Resuscitation,* **39,** 171–174.

Ruben, H. M., Elam, J. O. and Ruben, A. M. (1961) Investigation of upper airway problems in resuscitation. Studies of pharyngeal X-rays and performance by lay men. *Anesthesiology,* **22,** 271–279.

Ruge, J., Sinson, G., McLone, D. *et al.* (1988) Pediatric spinal injury: the very young. *J. Neurosurg.,* **68,** 25–30.

Ruppert, M., Reith, M., Widdman, J. *et al.* (1999) Checking for breathing: evaluation of the diagnostic capability of emergency medical services personnel, physicians, medical students and medical laypersons. *Ann. Emerg. Med.,* **34,** 720–729.

Safar, P. (1974) Pocket mask for emergency artificial ventilation and oxygen inhalation. *Crit. Care Med.,* **2,** 273–276.

Schilling, R. (1994) Should relatives witness resuscitation? *BMJ,* **309,** 406.

Schippel, P., Wild, L. and Burkhardt, U. (2001) Latex allergy in childhood – case reports. (German) *Anaesthesiolgie und Reanimation,* **26(4),** 105–108.

Schleien, C. L., Dean, J. M. and Koehler, R. C. (1986) Effect of epinephrine on cerebral and myocardial perfusion in an infant animal preparation of cardiopulmonary resuscitation. *Circulation,* **73,** 809–817.

Schnieder, S. (1992) Hypothermia: from recognition to rewarming. *Emerg. Med. Rep.,* **13,** 1–20.

Seigler, R. S., Tecklenburg, F. W. and Shealy, R. (1989) Prehospital intraosseous infusion by emergency medical services personnel: a prospective study. *Pediatrics,* **84,** 173–177.

Sellick, B. A. (1961) Cricoid pressure to control regurgitation of stomach contents during the induction of anaesthesia. *Lancet,* **2,** 404.

Shanon, M. and Liebelt, E. (1998) Targeted management strategies for cardiovascular toxicity from tricyclic antidepressant overdose: the pivotal role for alkalinisation and sodium loading. *Pediatr. Emerg. Care,* **14,** 293–298.

Sieber, F. and Traystman, R. (1992) Special issues: glucose and the brain. *Crit. Care Med.,* **20,** 104–114.

Siebke, H., Rod, T., Breivik, H. *et al.* (1975) Survival after 40 minutes; submersion without cerebral sequelae. *Lancet,* **1,** 1275–1277.

Simmons, C., Johnson, N., Perkin, R. *et al.* (1994) Intraosseous extravasation complication reports. *Ann. Emerg. Med.,* **23,** 363–366.

Simons, J. (1998) *Care of the Dying Child* (Goldman, A. ed). Oxford University Press, Oxford.

Simons, F., Roberts, J. and Gu, X. (1998) Epinephrine absorption in children with a history of anaphylaxis. *J. Allergy Clin. Immunol.,* **101,** 33–37.

Simons, F., Gu, X., Silver, N. *et al.* (2002) EpiPen Jr versus EpiPen in young children weighing 15–30kg at risk of anaphylaxis. *J. Allergy Clin. Immunol.,* **109,** 171–175.

Sirbaugh, P., Pepe, P., Shook, J. *et al.* (1999) A prospective, population-based study of the demographics, epidemiology, management, and outcome of out-of-hospital pediatric cardiopulmonary arrest. *Ann. Emerg. Med.,* **33,** 174–184.

Sirna, S. J., Ferguson, D. W., Charbonnier, F. *et al.* (1988) Factors affecting transthoracic impedence during electrical cardioversion. *Am. J. Cardiol.,* **62,** 1048–1052.

Skinner, D. and Vincent, R. (1997) *Cardiopulmonary Resuscitation,* 2nd edn. Oxford University Press, Oxford.

Smith, S. and Hatchett, R. (1992) Perceived competence in cardiopulmonary resuscitation, knowledge and skills among 50 qualified nurses. *Intens. Crit. Care Nurs.,* **8,** 76–81.

Southwick, F. and Dalglish, P. Jr. (1980) Recovery after prolonged asystolic cardiac arrest in profound hypothermia: a case report and literature review. *JAMA,* **243,** 1250–1253.

Spearpoint, K. (2002) National Audit of Paediatric Resuscitation (NAPR) presentation at Resuscitation Council (UK) Instructor's Day, April 11, Birmingham.

Steedman, D. and Robertson, C. (1992) Acid base changes in arterial and central venous blood during cardiopulmonary resuscitation. *Arch. Emerg. Med.,* **9,** 169–176.

Stewart, C. (2000) When lightning strikes. *Emerg. Med. Serv.,* **29(3),** 57–67, 103.

Stone, B., Chantler, P. and Baskett, P. (1998) The incidence of regurgitation during cardiopulmonary resuscitation: a comparison between the bag-valve-mask and laryngeal mask airway. *Resuscitation,* **38,** 3–6.

Stueven, H., Thompson, B., Aprahamian, C. *et al.* (1985a) Lack of effectiveness of calcium chloride in refractory asystole. *Ann. Emerg. Med.,* **14,** 630–632.

Stueven, H., Thompson, B., Aprahamian, C. *et al.* (1985b) Lack of effectiveness of calcium chloride in refractory electromechanical dissociation. *Ann. Emerg. Med.,* **14,** 626–629.

Tan, B., Sher, M., Good, R. *et al.* (2001) Severe food allergies by skin contact. *Ann. Allerg. Asthma Im.,* **86(5),** 583–586.

Teasdale, G. and Jennett, B. (1974) Assessment of coma and impaired consciousness: a practical scale. *Lancet,* **2,** 81–84.

Tendrup, T., Kanter, R. and Cherry, R. (1989) A comparison of infant ventilation methods performed by pre-hospital personnel. *Ann. Emerg. Med.,* **18,** 607–611.

Thompson, J. and Ashwal, S. (1983) Electrical injuries in children. *Am. J. Dis. Child.,* **137,** 231–235.

Tobias, J., Lynch, A. and Garrett, J. (1996) Alterations of end-tidal carbon dioxide during the intrahospital transport of children. *Pediatr. Emerg. Care,* **12,** 249–251.

Tonkin, S., Davis, S. and Gunn, T. (1995) Nasal route for infant resuscitation by mothers. *Lancet,* **345,** 1353–1354.

United Kingdom Central Council for Nursing, Midwifery, and Health Visiting (UKCC) (1998) *Guidelines for Records and Record Keeping.* UKCC, London.

Vidal, R., Kissoon, N. and Gayle, M. (1993) Compartment syndrome following intraosseous infusion. *Pediatrics, 91,* 1201–1202.

Wallace, J. (1991) Electrical injuries. In: *Harrison's Principles of Internal Medicine,* 12th edn (Fauci, A., Braunwald, E. and Isselbacher, K. eds). McGraw-Hill, New York.

Weil, M., Rackow, E., Trevino, R. *et al.* (1986) Difference in acid–base state between venous and arterial blood during cardiopulmonary resuscitation. *N. Eng. J. Med.,* **315,** 153–156.

Wenzel, V., Idris, A., Banner, M. *et al.* (1994) The composition of gas given by mouth-to-mouth ventilation during CPR. *Chest,* **106,** 1806–1810.

Whyte, S. and Wyllie, J. (1999) Paediatric life support: a practical assessment. *Resuscitation, 41,* 153–157.

Wittenborg, M., Gyepes, M. and Crocker, D. (1967) Tracheal dynamics in infants with respiratory distress, stridor, and collapsing trachea. *Radiology,* **88,** 653–662.

Wong, D., Hockenberry-Eaton, M., Wilson, D. *et al.* (1999) *Nursing Care of Infants and Children,* 6th edn. Mosby, London.

Wright, B. (1996) *Sudden Death. A Research Base for Practice,* 2nd edn. Churchill Livingstone, Edinburgh.

Wynne, G. (1995) Training and retention of skills. In: *ABC of Resuscitation* (Colquhoun, M., Handley, A. and Evans, T. eds). BMJ Books, London.

Wynne, G., Marteau, T., Johnson, M. *et al.* (1987) Inability of trained nurses to perform basic life support. *BMJ,* **284,** 1198–1199.

Young, K. and Seidel, J. (1999) Pediatric cardiopulmonary resuscitation: a collective review. *Ann. Emerg. Med.,* **33,** 195–205.

Zaritsky, A., Nadkarni, V., Getson, P. *et al.* (1987) CPR in children. *Ann. Emerg. Med.,* **16,** 1107–1111.

Zhou, X., Daubert, J., Wolf, P. *et al.* (1980) Size of the critical mass for defibrillation. Abstracts of the 62nd Scientific Session of the American Heart Association. *Circulation,* **80(Suppl 2),** 531.

Zideman, D. (1994) Resuscitation in infants and children. In: *ABC of Resuscitation* (Colquhoun, M. ed). BMJ, London.

Zideman, D. (1997) Paediatric resuscitation. In: *Cardiopulmonary Resuscitation,* 2nd edn (Skinner, D. and Vincent, R. eds). Oxford University Press, Oxford.

Zideman, D. and Spearpoint, K. (1999) Resuscitation of infants and children. In: *ABC of Resuscitation,* 4th edn (Colquhoun, M., Handley, A. and Evans, T. eds). BMJ Books, London.

Zoll, P. M., Linenthal, A. J. and Gibson, W. (1956) Termination of ventricular fibrillation in man by externally applied electric countershock. *N. Engl. J. Med.,* **254,** 727–732.

Zoltie, N., Sloan, J. and Wright, B. (1994) Observed resuscitation may affect a doctor's performance. *BMJ,* **309,** 406.

Index

Nursing and Midwifery Council (NMC
formerly UKCC) (*cont'd*)
Guidelines for records and record keeping
(UKCC/NMC) 143, 144, 154
Nursing staff
in reception of critically ill children
7–8
in retrieval of critically ill children
131–2

O

Oakley Chart 15
Opiate poisoning 116–17
Oropharyngeal airway 54–6
Outlet valve (of self-inflating bag) 66
Oxygen 88–9
in anaphylaxis 105
availability 15
delivery principles 62–8
saturation monitoring (incl. pulse
oximetry) 25
in post-resuscitation care 120
Oxygen inlet (of self-inflating bag) 66
Oxygen reservoir valve/bag 66–7, 68

P

P wave 71
Pacing, bradyarrhythmia 101
Paddles and pads, defibrillator
in automated external defibrillation
85
interface with skin 82
in manual defibrillation 84
position 83
pressure 82
size 81–2
in synchronized cardioversion 87
Paediatric ALS course (Resuscitation
Council) 160–1
Paediatric Glasgow Coma Scale 123,
124, 125
Paediatric Intensive Care Society
Standards Document
on general standards 9–10
on reception of child in hospital 7–9
on referral to paediatric ICU 128–30
Paediatric Life Support course (ALS
Group Manchester) 161
Paediatric Resuscitation and Emergency
Management System 16–18
Pallor with inadequate ventilation 25

Parasympathetic nervous system and
heart rate 71
Parents/family/relatives/carers 10
bereavement 135–42
in reception of critically ill children,
support for 7
resuscitation witnessed by 141–2
in retrieval of critically ill children
132
Patient outlet (of self-inflating bag) 66
Perfusion, tissue, poor, clinical signs 121
Photograph for bereaved family 140
Pneumothorax, tension 100
Pocket mask 32, 62–3
Poisoning (toxic drugs/chemicals) 100,
116–17
risk to staff 31
Polaroid photograph for bereaved
family 140
Police informed of death 138
Position of child indicating respiratory
problems 24–5
Post-mortem 138–9
Posture in neurological dysfunction 28
Potassium disturbances 100
PREM (Paediatric Resuscitation and
Emergency Management)
System 16–18
Pressure relief valve (of self-inflating
bag) 66
Protecting children from harm 10
Pulmonary embolism 101
Pulse, evaluation 26
in basic life support 35–6
in hypothermia 111
Pulse oximetry, *see* Oxygen
Pulseless electrical activity
(electromechanical dissociation)
2–3, 92
primary 2
secondary 3
Pulseless VT 2, 79
Pupillary response 28

Q

QRS complexes 71
rate/rhythm/width assessment 74

R

R waves in cardioversion 87
Records and documentation 143–6

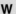